Controversies in Testosterone Deficiency

John P. Mulhall • Mario Maggi • Landon Trost
Editors

Controversies in Testosterone Deficiency

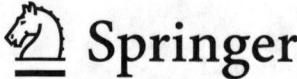 Springer

Editors
John P. Mulhall
Department of Urology
Memorial Sloan Kettering Cancer Center
New York, NY
USA

Landon Trost
Male Fertility and Peyronie's Clinic
Orem, UT
USA

Mario Maggi
Endocrinology
University of Firenze
Firenze
Firenze
Italy

ISBN 978-3-030-77113-3   ISBN 978-3-030-77111-9   (eBook)
https://doi.org/10.1007/978-3-030-77111-9

This Springer imprint is published by the registered company Springer Nature Switzerland AG
The registered company address is: Gewerbestrasse 11, 6330 Cham, Switzerland

Contents

Contributors

Robert E. Brannigan Northwestern University, Feinberg School of Medicine, Evanston, IL, USA

Bahman Chavoshan Department of Graduate Medical Education, St. Mary Medical Center, Long Beach, CA, USA

David Geffen School of Medicine, University of California, Los Angeles, Los Angeles, CA, USA

Sarah Cipriani Andrology, Women's Endocrinology and Gender Incongruence Unit, Department of Experimental, Clinical, and Biomedical Sciences "Mario Serio", University of Florence, Florence, Italy

Carlotta Cocchetti Andrology, Women's Endocrinology and Gender Incongruence Unit, Careggi University Hospital, Florence, Italy

Aakash P. Desai Division of Hematology, MayoClinic, Rochester, MN, USA

Alessandra Daphne Fisher Andrology, Women's Endocrinology and Gender Incongruence Unit, Careggi University Hospital, Florence, Italy

Ronald S. Go Division of Hematology, Department of Internal Medicine, Mayo Clinic, Rochester, MN, USA

O. Hasan Cook County Health, Chicago, IL, USA

M. Houlihan Mayo Clinic, Rochester, MN, USA

Ilpo Huhtaniemi Institute of Reproductive and Developmental Biology, Department of Metabolism, Digestion and Reproduction, Imperial College London, London, UK

T. Kohler Mayo Clinic, Rochester, MN, USA

Peter Y. Liu Division of Endocrinology, Department of Medicine, The Lundquist Institute at Harbor-UCLA Medical Center, Torrance, CA, USA

David Geffen School of Medicine, University of California, Los Angeles, Los Angeles, CA, USA

David Geffen School of Medicine at UCLA, Division of Endocrinology and Metabolism, Department of Medicine, Harbor UCLA Medical Center and Los Angeles Biomedical Research Institute, Torrance, CA, USA

Elisa Maseroli Andrology, Women's Endocrinology and Gender Incongruence Unit, Department of Experimental, Clinical, and Biomedical Sciences "Mario Serio", University of Florence, Florence, Italy

John P. Mulhall Department of Urology, Memorial Sloan Kettering Cancer Center, New York, NY, USA

Carolyn A. Salter Department of Urology, Memorial Sloan Kettering Cancer Center, New York, NY, USA

Ronald Swerdloff Division of Endocrinology, Department of Medicine, The Lundquist Institute at Harbor-UCLA Medical Center, Torrance, CA, USA

Landon Trost Male Fertility and Peyronie's Clinic, Orem, UT, USA

Linda Vignozzi Andrology, Women's Endocrinology and Gender Incongruence Unit, Department of Experimental, Clinical, and Biomedical Sciences "Mario Serio", University of Florence, Florence, Italy

Christina Wang Division of Endocrinology, Department of Medicine, The Lundquist Institute at Harbor-UCLA Medical Center, Torrance, CA, USA

Clinical and Translational Science Institute, Harbor–UCLA Medical Center and The Lundquist Institute, Torrance, CA, USA

Danya Waqfi Division of Endocrinology, Department of Medicine, The Lundquist Institute at Harbor-UCLA Medical Center, Torrance, CA, USA

D. Yang Mayo Clinic, Rochester, MN, USA

Fiona Yuen Division of Endocrinology, Department of Medicine, The Lundquist Institute at Harbor-UCLA Medical Center, Torrance, CA, USA

Chapter 1
What to Measure: Testosterone or Free Testosterone?

Christina Wang and Ronald Swerdloff

1.1 Why Serum Testosterone Is Necessary for the Diagnosis of Testosterone Deficiency?

Low serum testosterone (T) levels in adult men can lead to significant clinical symptoms and signs of testosterone deficiency (TD). These include sexual dysfunction, low energy and vitality, mood changes, sleep disturbances, loss of body hair, loss of muscle and bone mass, increased visceral fat, mild anemia, and, in more severe testosterone deficiency, small testes and infertility. In adolescent boys, TD presents as delayed sexual development, absence of axillary, pubic and facial hair, failure of the testes to increase in size, gynecomastia, and eunuchoidal proportions. The symptoms of testosterone deficiency are non-specific, and physical signs may not be clinically detectable in some older men with TD.

In addition, screening questionnaires to assess the symptoms of TD may be useful in large clinical studies; however, they have low specificity and are generally not useful in a clinic to diagnose an individual with TD [1–6]. Even with the use of screening questionnaire and symptoms of TD, the confirmation of TD must be based on the precise and accurate measurement of serum T concentrations [7, 8]. Because serum T can be transiently suppressed during acute illnesses, physical and mental stress, and intensive exercise, T should not be measured when these

C. Wang (✉)
Division of Endocrinology, Department of Medicine, The Lundquist Institute
at Harbor-UCLA Medical Center, Torrance, CA, USA

Clinical and Translational Science Institute, Harbor–UCLA Medical Center
and The Lundquist Institute, Torrance, CA, USA
e-mail: wang@lundquist.org

R. Swerdloff
Division of Endocrinology, Department of Medicine, The Lundquist Institute
at Harbor-UCLA Medical Center, Torrance, CA, USA
e-mail: swerdloff@lundquist.org

© Springer Nature Switzerland AG 2021
J. P. Mulhall et al. (eds.), *Controversies in Testosterone Deficiency*,
https://doi.org/10.1007/978-3-030-77111-9_1

Table 1.1 Common conditions that may affect serum testosterone concentration

Acute	Chronic
Acute medical illness	Aging
Emotional stress	Obesity
Intense physical activity	Metabolic syndrome
Medications	Diabetes
Acute sleep disorders	Chronic medical illnesses
	Eating disorders
	Obstructive sleep apnea
	Medications (opiates and glucocorticoids)

conditions are present. More importantly, T concentrations may decrease with obesity, age, metabolic syndrome and diabetes, sleep disorders, eating disorders, chronic kidney and liver disease, and chronic use of opiates and glucocorticoids (Table 1.1) [9–14]. Thus, it is important to ascertain the general health of the patient as treatment of some of these conditions may restore serum T to the reference range.

1.2 What Methods Should Be Used for Serum Testosterone Measurements?

Immunoassays are used for measuring serum testosterone concentrations. Several publications in the early 2000s demonstrated that immunoassays used in many clinical laboratories with automated platforms depend on reagents and reference ranges provided by the manufacturers. Some of these automated platform assays provide results that are precise but not accurate with significant bias when compared to the "gold standard" of steroid assays – liquid chromatography-tandem mass spectrometry (LC-MS/MS) [15–17]. These tests had passing scores in proficiency testing when compared to the same method but differed significantly when compared against each other. The T measurements at low concentrations, e.g., in women and children, were most unreliable, which led the Endocrine Society to issue a position statement that emphasized the following : (1) mass spectrometry has better accuracy and specificity and may be the method of choice for measuring testosterone concentrations at low levels; (2) the clinician should know the method and the reference ranges of their laboratories [18]; and (3) standardization programs focusing on accuracy should be implemented and updated reference ranges be established for men, women, and children [18–20]. The Center for Disease Control and Prevention (CDC) Laboratory Science Division took up this challenge and established the Hormone Standardization Program with T measurement as the first hormone to have harmonized assays [21–23]. The goal of the program is not to define which method a laboratory should use but to create "testosterone measurements traceable to one accuracy basis allowing measurements to be comparable across methods, time and location" [22]. To date, not only reference and research laboratories participate in the program but also manufacturers of automated platforms and mass spectrometers. The CDC also assisted the College of American Pathology (CAP) to

Table 1.2 Accuracy-based testing of serum testosterone (ng/dL) from the College of American Pathologist 2020

	No. labs	Mean	SD	CV%	Median	Low	High
ABS-06 Method							
All	*68*	*494*	*58*	*11.8*	*499*	*356*	*628*
Abbott Architect	13	537	27	5.1	531	501	574
Beckman Unicel Dxl	7				426	382	446
Mass spectrometry	20	484	35	7.2	483	423	578
Roche Cobas e600	6				500	487	514
Roche Cobas e801	7				508	496	524
Siemens Advia Centaur XP/XPT	4				549	481	628
CDC reference method		460					
ABS-05 method							
All	*64*	*21.8*	*5.4*	*24.6*	*22*	*8*	*37*
Abbott Architect	13	25.3	2.5	10.0	25	20	29
Beckman Unicel Dxl	7				25	17	37
Mass spectrometry	20	21.9	2.8	12.7	22	12	26
Roche Cobas e600	6				16	13	17
Roche Cobas e801	7				15	12	17
Siemens Advia Centaur XP/XPT	4				25	24	32
CDC reference method		22.7					

introduce accuracy-based proficiency test for T assays with the participation of many clinical laboratories [24]. The results of the accuracy-based harmonization of T assays showed that with time (3.5 year) there was improvement in proficiency scores of both accuracy and precision in 65 participating clinical laboratories in State of New York [25]. The conclusion is that most clinical laboratories using automated platforms are aware that accuracy-based proficient testing should be implemented with improvement in the quality of the assay. The accuracy-based tests in recent CAP report showed very small difference within a method and between methods (Table 1.2). For the diagnosis and monitoring of T-replacement therapy in TD men, both immunoassay and LC-MS/MS methods are sufficient as the goal is to distinguish low concentrations from the population reference ranges of adult men. As shown in Table 1.2, with participation in accuracy-based external quality control, even low levels of testosterone showed good agreement within a method and between methods.

1.3   What Is the Reference Range for Serum Total Testosterone in Adult Men?

The generally accepted range of serum testosterone in adult men is 300–1000 ng/dL (10.4–34.7 nmol/L) based on immunoassays with a purification step before immunoassays [26]. There are many possible physiological explanations why men would have such a large range of testosterone levels. Once a standardized method has been validated [22], reference ranges can be established based on cross calibrating assays to a reference method. Using data from four population-based studies in Europe and the United States (1656 younger community-dwelling men in the Framingham Heart Study; European Male Aging Study; Osteoporotic Fractures in Men Study; and Male Sibling Study of Osteoporosis), the harmonized serum testosterone reference range (2.5th to 97.5th percentile) for non-obese men between 19 and 39 years was established to be between 264 and 916 ng/dL (9.16 to 31.8 nmol/L) [27]. Most of these men identified themselves as white and it should be noted that geographical and ethnic/racial differences in sex hormone levels have been reported in some studies [28–30]. Population-based studies of harmonized T levels in other ethnic/racial group have not yet been reported.

1.4   What Are the Precautions to Reduce the Variability in Serum Testosterone Concentrations?

Serum T concentrations should be measured from a blood sample collected early in the morning between 7 am and 10 am. The diurnal variation of serum T results in T levels higher in the early morning than later in the day in both young and middle-aged men [31]. This diurnal variation is attenuated in older men [32]. Most laboratories establish reference ranges for healthy adult men based on morning samples. Thus, to compare a patient with possible TD, blood samples should be drawn in the morning between 7 am and 10 am. There are data showing that acute ingestion of glucose lowers serum total testosterone by 25% [33]. Thus, for diagnosis of TD, it is important to obtain a fasting morning blood sample. In general, serum samples should be used for assays. Because T concentrations are affected by acute illnesses, mental and physical stress, and medications, a repeat morning T concentration provides confirmatory evidence that the low T level is probably persistent. It should be noted that after oral testosterone undecanoate administration, the high levels of testosterone undecanoate in blood can be cleaved by non-specific esterases ex vivo, so a blood collection tube with inhibitors of non-specific esterases (plasma) [34] should be used or more conveniently a conversion factor (serum T = plasma T/1.2) be applied to calculate serum T concentrations [35].

Accurate and precise measurement of serum testosterone is adequate for the diagnosis and monitoring of testosterone replacement for most men with TD. Serum testosterone measurement should be obtained in the morning, preferably in fasting state, and a repeat sample for confirmation is advisable. The sample should be sent to a reliable laboratory that practices accuracy-based proficiency tests or external quality control programs and quotes a reference range of serum testosterone levels of adult men between 250 and 1000 ng/dL (8.7 to 34.7 nmol/L).

1.5   What Is Free Testosterone?

In men, T and estradiol circulate bound tightly to the sex hormone binding globulin (SHBG) and loosely to albumin, and they also circulate in free or unbound form. This led to the free hormone hypothesis postulating that free and the loosely bound testosterone or estradiol can freely diffuse out to the capillaries into the cells of the target tissues to initiate appropriate responses to these sex hormones [36]. SHBG is a glycoprotein synthesized in the liver with high-affinity binding sites for T and estradiol [37, 38]. In men, about 50–55% of testosterone is bound to SHBG and the rest to albumin (45–48%), and the fraction of free testosterone is <2%. SHBG concentrations are affected by a number of factors (Table 1.3) [39]. Androgens (testosterone and its esters) and androgenic progestins (levonorgestrel, desogestrel, and progestins commonly used in female contraceptive pills) decrease SHBG levels. SHBG concentration is a good biomarker for androgen activity in the body. TD men have higher SHBG concentrations which decrease with androgen treatment. Since total T concentration is a measure of both bound and free testosterone, conditions where SHBG may be increased or decreased will affect the total T concentration. It is under these conditions that measurement of free T concentrations may be warranted (Table 1.3) [39]. For example, in an older overweight man with some symptoms of TD, aging increases and obesity decreases SHBG; in such circumstances, thus, to assess whether the older man has TD, measurement of serum free T may be indicated. Free T measurements may also be helpful in symptomatic men with borderline low T concentrations, e.g., between 250 and 350 ng/dL (8.7–12.2 nmol/L) [7]. The binding of T to SHBG is complex, which results in many different methods that directly measure or calculate free T. Some of these methods do not measure free fraction of T and some formulae may provide less accurate results [40].

Table 1.3 Factors that affect SHBG concentrations

Increase SHBG	Decrease SHBG
Estrogens	Androgens
Male hypogonadism	Androgenic progestins
Thyroid hormone, hyperthyroidism	Hypothyroidism
Pregnancy	Obesity, metabolic syndrome, type 2 diabetes
Aging	Hyperprolactinemia
Anticonvulsants	Acromegaly
Rifampin	Nephrotic syndrome
Alcoholic liver disease	End-stage liver disease

1.6   Are There Reliable Methods to Estimate Free Testosterone Concentrations?

The different methods of estimating free testosterone are shown in Table 1.4.

1.6.1   Free Testosterone by Equilibrium Dialysis

Free T can be measured by equilibrium dialysis where test serum or plasma is mixed with isotope-labeled T and dialyzed overnight into buffer solution. The free non-protein-bound fraction of the labeled T outside of the dialysis cell is the active "free fraction" of T. The free fraction (percent free T, usually between 1 to 2%) is multiplied by the total T measured by a reliable method to provide the free T concentration [41, 42]. This gold standard method of measuring free T by equilibrium dialysis is not automated, is cumbersome, and requires technical skill. Equilibrium dialysis methods are too complex for use in routine clinical chemistry laboratories. The methods are not harmonized and thus there are no common reference intervals to help clinicians to interpret free T concentrations [44]. Using this method, it has been found that concentrations of free T are normal even when the total testosterone is low in clinical conditions such as obesity [43] and other circumstances where SHBG is abnormal. Ultrafiltration methods are simpler but are sensitive to temperature changes, and difficult to standardize with reproducible data, and, therefore, are not commonly utilized today [45]. Recent studies

Table 1.4 Methods to measure serum free testosterone

Method	Advantages	Potential problems
Equilibrium dialysis	Gold standard to measure free testosterone	Not automated, required technical skills Require accurate testosterone assay Higher variability
Bioavailable testosterone	Technically easier	Not automated Require accurate testosterone assay
Salivary testosterone	Technically easy Does not require a blood draw	Collection issues may influence results
Calculated free testosterone	Can be automated Technically easy	Require accurate testosterone and SHBG assays Different formulae. Different algorithms may be better for different clinical questions
Analog free testosterone	Can be automated Technically easy	Does not measure free T Values are 1/5 of that from equilibrium dialysis Provides no additional information than total testosterone Recommend not to be used

indicate that the method has better consistency in some laboratories, and their usefulness as a modified methodology will need further validation across laboratories [46, 47].

1.6.2   Bioavailable Testosterone

The concept of bioavailable T is based on the theory that the free fraction and the loosely albumin-bound fraction of circulating T are available to the target organs and tissues [48]. Thus, not only the free but also the albumin-bound T is biologically active in tissues. Bioavailable T – the sum of albumin-bound and free testosterone – is generally measured in the serum after adding saturated ammonium sulfate solution to precipitate the SHBG-bound fraction. The separation of SHBG-bound testosterone can also be done by adding concanavalin A [49]. These methods are not automated and standardized and thus not generally available in routine laboratories but are available in reference laboratories [44]. These methods require accurate and precise measurment of T in the non-SHBG bound fraction after ammonium sulfate precipitation or ultracentrigfugation. Measurement of bioavailable T may be useful in men whose SHBG binding or concentration may be abnormal such as in older [50] and obese men [50].In most men with TD, measurement of bioavailable T is not usually required for diagnosis [51].

1.6.3   Salivary Testosterone

Because saliva does not contain SHBG, salivary T has been used as a surrogate for serum-free T [52, 53]. Salivary T can be measured by immunoassays or LC-MS/MS [54]. The concentration of T in the saliva may be influenced by the flow and also presence of blood in the sample. For these reasons and non-familiarity of use of saliva as a matrix, this simple method is not commonly used for free T determinations [55]; exceptions include the use of salivary T in studies on athletes and pre-pubertal children and infants where a blood draw can be avoided [56–58].

1.6.4   Calculated Free and Bioavailable Testosterone

Because of the technical difficulty, lack of automation, and absence of reference intervals for free T measured by equilibrium dialysis and bioavailable testosterone measured by ammonium sulfate precipitation methodologies (described above), these methods may not be suitable nor available in most routine clinical chemistry laboratories. This creates a widely utilized niche for calculated free T determinations. Calculated free and bioavailable T can be determined by using accurate and precise assays of T and SHBG [50, 59, 60]. Using different equations/algorithms, both free and bioavailable T may be calculated [59, 60], which have been recommended as suitable for routine clinical use [18, 44, 59]. The most commonly used equations based on the law of mass action [41, 60–62] are used to calculate both the free and bioavailable T. Other investigators have recommended the use of empirically derived equations that fitted the clinical populations studied [63, 64]; but these empirical equations are not widely used. The calculated free T using law of mass action formula overestimates free T measured by equilibrium dialysis. Empirical formulae are free from assumptions and may be more concordant with the measured free T [63]. Recent evidence suggests that the law of mass action formula which is based on the assumption that two T molecules bind to two binding sites on the SHBG with similar binding affinity may be incorrect. And further argues that the binding of T to SHBG may be a multistep, dynamic process with complex allosteric characteristics [65]. Based on this new model, investigators used a new formula to calculate free T in younger men in the Framingham Heart study and showed that the newly calculated values were similar to those measured by equilibrium dialysis. They further verified that the calculated free T values had clinical diagnostic validity using data from the European Male Aging Study. They demonstrated that men with calculated free T below the reference range had higher risk of sexual symptoms and elevated LH suggestive of primary TD. While enticing, the use of this new formula must be further validated by other laboratories. The Endocrine Society suggests that calculated free T may be the most practical method to measure free T using accuracy and precise total T and SHBG measurements [7, 18]. Currently the CDC is developing a harmonized method for free T based on calculated free T using revised formulae. This may bring the measurement of free T to a referable standard in clinical laboratories and common reference intervals that all clinicians can use.

1.6.5   Analog-Based Immunoassays and Why They Are Not Recommended by Most Experts in the Field

Analog-based free T assaysare offered by most clinical laboratories, are measured on automated platforms, and are widely used by clinicians. However, many studies have shown that free T concentrations measured by analog-based immunoassay are about one-fifth the concentrations measured by equilibrium dialysis and are related to SHBG [59, 66] or total T concentration [67] and do not reflect free T concentrations in clinical conditions such as hirsutism and hyperthyroidism [18, 68]. Experiments using varying concentrations of SHBG and T showed that analog-based free T immunoassay reported free T results that were related primarily to total T and concluded that free T analog assays do not detect serum free T [67]. Some argue that free T concentrations measured by immunoassays are as good as calculated free T but failed to note that the free T values obtained by immunoassays are only 1/7 of those measured by equilibrium dialysis indicating clearly what is measured by the analog free T assays is not free T [69]. The Endocrine Society Position Statement indicates that analog-based assays have poor accuracy, sensitivity, and poor correlation with equilibrium dialysis method [18]. Free T by analog immunoassay correlates with total serum T and provides no additional information and is not a measure of free T and should not be used.

1.7   Does Measurement of Free Testosterone Provide Additional Information for Clinical Diagnosis?

In most instances for the diagnosis of TD, total T measured in the morning should suffice if the concentrations are repeatedly below the reference range of the laboratory. In circumstances where concentration of serum SHBG may be affected by liver or kidney disease, thyroid dysfunction, or other endocrine disorders (Table 1.3), the measurement of free T either calculated or by equilibrium dialysis may be warranted. For most clinicians, free T may be useful when older, overweight men with some symptoms suggestive of TD have serum T concentrations in the borderline range (e.g., between 250 and 350 ng/dL or 8.7 and 12.2 nmol/L). Aging is associated with a decrease in total serum T levels and an increase in SHBG, resulting in a greater decrease in free T, provided men are not obese. This is because obesity results in lower SHBG and lower total T, but the free testosterone concentration may be normal [43]. In a large population-based study (European Male Aging Study, 3349 men aged 40–79 years), men with normal total but low calculated free T were older with poorer health and exhibited more sexual symptoms, whereas those with low total T and normal free T were more obese and had no features of androgen deficiency. The results suggested that older men with lower free T have symptoms suggestive of androgen deficiency, despite having normal total T levels [70]. Furthermore compared to older obese men with low total T and normal or low luteinizing hormone (LH), men who have low free T had more sexual symptoms including lower sexual desire and infrequent morning erections, which suggests that low free T may be indicative of symptomatic TD [71]. The Testosterone Trials in which older men with symptomatic TD were administered placebo or T gel daily for a year showed that baseline total and free T were significantly and independently associated with sexual desire, erectile function, and sexual activity but not with vitality or physical function [72]. In addition, after treatment with T gel, the improvements in sexual activity and desire were associated with both serum total T and free TD, indicating that the sexual function improvement was related to the incremental increases of both serum total T and free T [73]. These studies indicate that in older men with symptoms suggestive of TD, measurement of free T may be indicated even when total T concentration may be normal. Perhaps the newer formula for calculated free T validated in multiple laboratories [65], will become generally available, correlate with free T by equilibrium dialysis and demonstrate improved correlation with clinical symptoms and therapeutic responsiveness. If all these prove to be true, then this formula to calculate free T may be a justified replacement for free T measurement by the equilibrium dialysis methodology.

Diagnosis of symptomatic TD relies principally on measurement of total testosterone. Free testosterone may provide additional information if there are issues with the concentration or the binding of testosterone to SHBG. Free testosterone should be measured by equilibrium dialysis which is available in reference laboratories or by calculated free testosterone using formulae that have been validated and accurate and precise measurements of both testosterone and SHBG. The most common clinical use of free testosterone is for the diagnosis of hypogonadism of older men who may be overweight.

References

Uncategorized References

1. Heinemann LAJ, Zimmermann T, Vermeulen A, et al. A new "aging males" symptoms' rating scale. Aging Male. 1999;2:105–14.
2. Morley JE, Charlton E, Patrick P, et al. Validation of a screening questionnaire for androgen deficiency in aging males. Metabolism. 2000;49(9):1239–42.
3. Smith KW, Feldman HA, McKinlay JB. Construction and field validation of a self-administered screener for testosterone deficiency (hypogonadism) in ageing men. Clin Endocrinol. 2000;53(6):703–11.
4. Rosen RC, Araujo AB, Connor MK, et al. Assessing symptoms of hypogonadism by self-administered questionnaire: qualitative findings in patients and controls. Aging Male. 2009;12(2–3):77–85.
5. Rosen RC, Araujo AB, Connor MK, et al. The NERI Hypogonadism Screener: psychometric validation in male patients and controls. Clin Endocrinol. 2011;74(2):248–56.
6. Heinemann LA, Saad F, Heinemann K, et al. Can results of the Aging Males' Symptoms (AMS) scale predict those of screening scales for androgen deficiency? Aging Male. 2004;7(3):211–8.
7. Bhasin S, Brito JP, Cunningham GR, et al. Testosterone therapy in men with hypogonadism: an Endocrine Society clinical practice guideline. J Clin Endocrinol Metab. 2018;103(5):1715–44.
8. Matsumoto AM, Bremner WJ. Serum testosterone assays – accuracy matters. J Clin Endocrinol Metab. 2004;89(2):520–4.
9. Corona G, Monami M, Rastrelli G, et al. Type 2 diabetes mellitus and testosterone: a meta-analysis study. Int J Androl. 2010;34:528–40.
10. Araujo AB, O'Donnell AB, Brambilla DJ, et al. Prevalence and incidence of androgen deficiency in middle-aged and older men: estimates from the Massachusetts Male Aging Study. J Clin Endocrinol Metab. 2004;89(12):5920–6.
11. Harman SM, Metter EJ, Tobin JD, et al. Longitudinal effects of aging on serum total and free testosterone levels in healthy men. Baltimore Longitudinal Study of Aging. J Clin Endocrinol Metab. 2001;86(2):724–31.
12. Wu FC, Tajar A, Beynon JM, et al. Identification of late-onset hypogonadism in middle-aged and elderly men. N Engl J Med. 2010;363(2):123–35.
13. Bercea RM, Mihaescu T, Cojocaru C, et al. Fatigue and serum testosterone in obstructive sleep apnea patients. Clin Respir J. 2015;9(3):342–9.

14. Clarke BM, Vincent AD, Martin S, et al. Obstructive sleep apnea is not an independent determinant of testosterone in men. Eur J Endocrinol. 2020;183(1):31–9.
15. Wang C, Catlin DH, Demers LM, et al. Measurement of total serum testosterone in adult men: comparison of current laboratory methods versus liquid chromatography-tandem mass spectrometry. J Clin Endocrinol Metab. 2004;89(2):534–43.
16. Taieb J, Mathian B, Millot F, et al. Testosterone measured by 10 immunoassays and by isotope-dilution gas chromatography-mass spectrometry in sera from 116 men, women, and children. Clin Chem. 2003;49(8):1381–95.
17. Sikaris K, McLachlan RI, Kazlauskas R, et al. Reproductive hormone reference intervals for healthy fertile young men: evaluation of automated platform assays. J Clin Endocrinol Metab. 2005;90(11):5928–36.
18. Rosner W, Auchus RJ, Azziz R, et al. Position statement: utility, limitations, and pitfalls in measuring testosterone: an Endocrine Society position statement. J Clin Endocrinol Metab. 2007;92(2):405–13.
19. Rosner W, Vesper H. Preface. CDC workshop report improving steroid hormone measurements in patient care and research translation. Steroids. 2008;73(13):1285.
20. Rosner W, Vesper H. Toward excellence in testosterone testing: a consensus statement. J Clin Endocrinol Metab. 2010;95(10):4542–8.
21. Vesper HW, Bhasin S, Wang C, et al. Interlaboratory comparison study of serum total testosterone measurements performed by mass spectrometry methods. Steroids. 2009;74(6):498–503.
22. Vesper HW, Botelho JC. Standardization of testosterone measurements in humans. J Steroid Biochem Mol Biol. 2010;121(3–5):513–9.
23. Vesper HW, Botelho JC, Shacklady C, et al. CDC project on standardizing steroid hormone measurements. Steroids. 2008;73(13):1286–92.
24. Cao ZT, Botelho JC, Rej R, et al. Accuracy-based proficiency testing for testosterone measurements with immunoassays and liquid chromatography-mass spectrometry. Clin Chim Acta. 2017;469:31–6.
25. Cao ZT, Botelho JC, Rej R, et al. Impact of testosterone assay standardization efforts assessed via accuracy-based proficiency testing. Clin Biochem. 2019;68:37–43.
26. Griffin PD, Wilson JD. Disorders of the testis. In: Braunwald E, Fauci AS, Kasper DL, Hauser SL, Longo DL, Jamieson JL, editors. Harrison's principles of internal medicine. 15th ed. New York: MaGraw Hill; 2001. p. 2143–54.
27. Travison TG, Vesper HW, Orwoll E, et al. Harmonized reference ranges for circulating testosterone levels in men of four cohort studies in the United States and Europe. J Clin Endocrinol Metab. 2017;102(4):1161–73.
28. Orwoll ES, Nielson CM, Labrie F, et al. Evidence for geographical and racial variation in serum sex steroid levels in older men. J Clin Endocrinol Metab. 2010;95(10):E151–E60.
29. Vesper HW, Wang Y, Vidal M, et al. Serum total testosterone concentrations in the US household population from the NHANES 2011–2012 study population. Clin Chem. 2015;61(12):1495–504.
30. Litman HJ, Bhasin S, Link CL, et al. Serum androgen levels in black, Hispanic, and white men. J Clin Endocrinol Metab. 2006;91(11):4326–34.
31. Diver MJ, Imtiaz KE, Ahmad AM, et al. Diurnal rhythms of serum total, free and bioavailable testosterone and of SHBG in middle-aged men compared with those in young men. Clin Endocrinol. 2003;58(6):710–7.
32. Bremner WJ, Vitiello MV, Prinz PN. Loss of circadian rhythmicity in blood testosterone levels with aging in normal men. J Clin Endocrinol Metab. 1983;56(6):1278–81.
33. Caronia LM, Dwyer AA, Hayden D, et al. Abrupt decrease in serum testosterone levels after an oral glucose load in men: implications for screening for hypogonadism. Clin Endocrinol. 2013;78(2):291–6.
34. Ceponis J, Swerdloff R, Leung A, et al. Accurate measurement of androgen after androgen esters: problems created by ex vivo esterase effects and LC-MS/MS interference. Andrology. 2019;7(1):42–52.

35. Swerdloff RS, Wang C, White WB, et al. A new oral testosterone undecanoate formulation restores testosterone to normal concentrations in hypogonadal men. J Clin Endocrinol Metab. 2020;105(8):2515–31.
36. Pardridge WM. Serum bioavailability of sex steroid hormones. Clin Endocrinol Metab. 1986;15(2):259–78.
37. Iqbal MJ, Johnson MW. Purification and characterization of human sex hormone binding globulin. J Steroid Biochem. 1979;10(5):535–40.
38. Rosner W, Smith RN. Isolation and characterization of the testosterone-estradiol-binding globulin from human plasma. Use of a novel affinity column. Biochemistry (Mosc). 1975;14(22):4813–20.
39. Selby C. Sex hormone binding globulin: origin, function and clinical significance. Ann Clin Biochem. 1990;27(Pt 6):532–41.
40. Goldman AL, Bhasin S, Wu FCW, et al. A reappraisal of testosterone's binding in circulation: physiological and clinical implications. Endocr Rev. 2017;38(4):302–24.
41. Vermeulen A, Stoica T, Verdonck L. The apparent free testosterone concentration, an index of androgenicity. J Clin Endocrinol Metab. 1971;33(5):759–67.
42. Kley HK, Bartmann E, Krüskemper HL. A simple and rapid method to measure non-protein-bound fractions of cortisol, testosterone and oestradiol by equilibrium dialysis: comparison with centrifugal filtration. Acta Endocrinol. 1977;85(1):209–19.
43. Glass AR, Swerdloff RS, Bray GA, et al. Low serum testosterone and sex-hormone-binding-globulin in massively obese men. J Clin Endocrinol Metab. 1977;45(6):1211–9.
44. Keevil BG, Adaway J. Assessment of free testosterone concentration. J Steroid Biochem Mol Biol. 2019;190:207–11.
45. Hammond GL, Nisker JA, Jones LA, et al. Estimation of the percentage of free steroid in undiluted serum by centrifugal ultrafiltration-dialysis. J Biol Chem. 1980;255(11):5023–6.
46. Chen Y, Yazdanpanah M, Wang XY, et al. Direct measurement of serum free testosterone by ultrafiltration followed by liquid chromatography tandem mass spectrometry. Clin Biochem. 2010;43(4–5):490–6.
47. Van Uytfanghe K, Stöckl D, Kaufman JM, et al. Validation of 5 routine assays for serum free testosterone with a candidate reference measurement procedure based on ultrafiltration and isotope dilution-gas chromatography-mass spectrometry. Clin Biochem. 2005;38(3):253–61.
48. Manni A, Pardridge WM, Cefalu W, et al. Bioavailability of albumin-bound testosterone. J Clin Endocrinol Metab. 1985;61(4):705–10.
49. Giton F, Guéchot J, Fiet J. Comparative determinations of non SHBG-bound serum testosterone, using ammonium sulfate precipitation, Concanavalin A binding or calculation in men. Steroids. 2012;77(12):1306–11.
50. Fabbri E, An Y, Gonzalez-Freire M, et al. Bioavailable testosterone linearly declines over a wide age spectrum in men and women from the Baltimore Longitudinal Study of Aging. J Gerontol A Biol Sci Med Sci. 2016;71(9):1202–9.
51. Gheorghiu I, Moshyk A, Lepage R, et al. When is bioavailable testosterone a redundant test in the diagnosis of hypogonadism in men? Clin Biochem. 2005;38(9):813–8.
52. Wang C, Plymate S, Nieschlag E, et al. Salivary testosterone in men: further evidence of a direct correlation with free serum testosterone. J Clin Endocrinol Metab. 1981;53(5):1021–4.
53. Fiers T, Kaufman JM. Management of hypogonadism: is there a role for salivary testosterone. Endocrine. 2015;50(1):1–3.
54. Büttler RM, Peper JS, Crone EA, et al. Reference values for salivary testosterone in adolescent boys and girls determined using Isotope-Dilution Liquid-Chromatography Tandem Mass Spectrometry (ID-LC-MS/MS). Clin Chim Acta. 2016;456:15–8.
55. Granger DA, Shirtcliff EA, Booth A, et al. The "trouble" with salivary testosterone. Psychoneuroendocrinology. 2004;29(10):1229–40.
56. Contreras M, Raisingani M, Chandler DW, et al. Salivary testosterone during the minipuberty of infancy. Horm Res Paediatr. 2017;87(2):111–5.

57. de Arruda AFS, Aoki MS, Drago G, et al. Salivary testosterone concentration, anxiety, per-
    ceived performance and ratings of perceived exertion in basketball players during semi-final
    and final matches. Physiol Behav. 2019;198:102–7.
58. Hayes LD, Sculthorpe N, Cunniffe B, et al. Salivary testosterone and cortisol measurement
    in sports medicine: a narrative review and user's guide for researchers and practitioners. Int J
    Sports Med. 2016;37(13):1007–18.
59. Vermeulen A, Verdonck L, Kaufman JM. A critical evaluation of simple methods for the esti-
    mation of free testosterone in serum. J Clin Endocrinol Metab. 1999;84(10):3666–72.
60. Sodergard R, Backstrom T, Shanbhag V, et al. Calculation of free and bound fractions of
    testosterone and estradiol-17 beta to human plasma proteins at body temperature. J Steroid
    Biochem. 1982;16(6):801–10.
61. Mazer NA. A novel spreadsheet method for calculating the free serum concentrations of tes-
    tosterone, dihydrotestosterone, estradiol, estrone and cortisol: with illustrative examples from
    male and female populations. Steroids. 2009;74(6):512–9.
62. Nanjee MN, Wheeler MJ. Plasma free testosterone--is an index sufficient? Ann Clin Biochem.
    1985;22(Pt 4):387–90.
63. Ly LP, Sartorius G, Hull L, et al. Accuracy of calculated free testosterone formulae in men.
    Clin Endocrinol. 2010;73:382–8.
64. Sartorius G, Ly LP, Sikaris K, et al. Predictive accuracy and sources of variability in calculated
    free testosterone estimates. Ann Clin Biochem. 2009;46(Pt 2):137–43.
65. Zakharov MN, Bhasin S, Travison TG, et al. A multi-step, dynamic allosteric model of testos-
    terone's binding to sex hormone binding globulin. Mol Cell Endocrinol. 2015;399:190–200.
66. Winters SJ, Kelley DE, Goodpaster B. The analog free testosterone assay: are the results in
    men clinically useful? Clin Chem. 1998;44(10):2178–82.
67. Fritz KS, McKean AJ, Nelson JC, et al. Analog-based free testosterone test results linked
    to total testosterone concentrations, not free testosterone concentrations. Clin Chem.
    2008;54(3):512–6.
68. Rosner W. An extraordinarily inaccurate assay for free testosterone is still with us. J Clin
    Endocrinol Metab. 2001;86(6):2903.
69. Kacker R, Hornstein A, Morgentaler A. Free testosterone by direct and calculated measure-
    ment versus equilibrium dialysis in a clinical population. Aging Male. 2013;16(4):164–8.
70. Antonio L, Wu FC, O'Neill TW, et al. Low free testosterone is associated with hypogo-
    nadal signs and symptoms in men with normal total testosterone. J Clin Endocrinol Metab.
    2016;101(7):2647–57.
71. Rastrelli G, O'Neill TW, Ahern T, et al. Symptomatic androgen deficiency develops only
    when both total and free testosterone decline in obese men who may have incident bio-
    chemical secondary hypogonadism: prospective results from the EMAS. Clin Endocrinol.
    2018;89(4):459–69.
72. Cunningham GR, Stephens-Shields AJ, Rosen RC, et al. Association of sex hormones with
    sexual function, vitality, and physical function of symptomatic older men with low testosterone
    levels at baseline in the testosterone trials. J Clin Endocrinol Metab. 2015;100(3):1146–55.
73. Cunningham GR, Stephens-Shields AJ, Rosen RC, et al. Testosterone treatment and
    sexual function in older men with low testosterone levels. J Clin Endocrinol Metab.
    2016;101(8):3096–104.

Chapter 2
Erythrocytosis in Patients on Testosterone Therapy

Aakash P. Desai and Ronald S. Go

2.1   Introduction

With increasing awareness of men's health and related issues, in particular androgen deficiency, there has been a rise in the use of testosterone therapy. Prescription sales of testosterone have nearly tripled between 2001 and 2011 [1]. Various formulations of testosterone therapy have evolved over time including gels, pellets, injections, and, more recently, oral formulations. Testosterone therapy is largely used for testosterone deficiency. Studies have found that the prevalence of testosterone deficiency varies from 23% to 38% as men age [2, 3]. Testosterone levels <300 ng/dl in men are considered low. Despite this, most professional society guidelines recommend treatment only in men with concomitant hypogonadal symptoms [4]. This is due to the potential side effects of testosterone therapy including, but not limited to, increased estrogen levels, gynecomastia, erythrocytosis, thrombosis, and prostate cancer [5]. This chapter will discuss erythrocytosis in the context of testosterone replacement therapy.

2.2   Definition of Erythrocytosis

Erythrocytosis refers to increased concentration of erythrocytes in the blood. It essentially includes increase in the number of red blood cells (RBCs), hemoglobin level, or hematocrit. This phenomenon may also be due to a reduction in plasma

A. P. Desai
Division of Hematology, MayoClinic, Rochester, MN, USA

R. S. Go (✉)
Division of Hematology, Department of Internal Medicine, Mayo Clinic,
Rochester, MN, USA
e-mail: Go.Ronald@mayo.edu

© Springer Nature Switzerland AG 2021
J. P. Mulhall et al. (eds.), *Controversies in Testosterone Deficiency*,
https://doi.org/10.1007/978-3-030-77111-9_2

volume [6]. Polycythemia, a term often used interchangeably with erythrocytosis, is defined as an increase in the RBC volume or mass and generally refers to polycythemia vera. Typically, hematologists use erythrocytosis to describe an increase in hemoglobin (Hgb) or hematocrit (Hct) and reserve the word polycythemia for polycythemia vera. Although "erythrocytosis" is commonly used by the British Society of Hematology, the American Society of Hematology, and the World Health Organization classification, it is still not uniformly used across various specialties.

The normal levels of hemoglobin are 13.5–17.5 g/dL and 12–16 g/dL and the normal levels of hematocrit are 41–51% and 36–46% in males and females, respectively [7].

2.3   Rates of Erythrocytosis During Testosterone Therapy

Various studies have demonstrated the rate of developing erythrocytosis while on testosterone therapy to be around 0.8–6% depending on the dose used and the duration of treatment (Table 2.1) [8–12]. In a meta-analysis of three placebo-controlled clinical trials, which enrolled a total of 1579 participants, the relative risk of erythrocytosis was 8.14 (1.87–35.40) in the testosterone arms compared with the placebo arms [10]. Testosterone therapy causes erythrocytosis through various mechanisms which include elevation of erythropoietin and suppression of hepcidin, which subsequently results in increased iron absorption, increased systemic iron transport, and erythropoiesis [13]. Most clinical trials use hemoglobin of 17.5 g/dl and

Table 2.1 Studies demonstrating prevalence of erythrocytosis in testosterone therapy

Study (year)	Study duration	Preparations	Sample size	Hct > 54%	Comments
Snyder et al. (2016) [11]	12 months	T gel 1% 5 g QD initially	394	1.8%	Age > 65 years; dose adjusted at mos. 1,2,3,6,9 to T level
		Placebo	394	0%	
Brock et al. (2016) [8]	12 weeks	T solution 2% 60 mg QD	358	1.8%	Age > 18 years; dose adjusted at wks. 4 and 8 per T level
		Placebo	357	0.3%	
Paduch et al. (2015) [9]	16 weeks	T solution 2% 60 mg QD	36	0.8%	Age ≥ 26 years; dose adjusted at wks. 4 per T level
		Placebo	40	0%	
Steidle et al. (2003) [12]	13 weeks	T gel 1% 50 mg QD	99	3%	Age > 20 years; dose adjusted at day 60 per T level
		T gel 1% 100 mg QD	106	6%	
		T patch 5 mg QD	102	1%	
		Placebo	99	1%	

Abbreviations: *T* testosterone, *QD* daily, *wks* weeks

hematocrit of 54% as definition of erythrocytosis. However, Endocrine Society guidelines recommend using a hematocrit >50% as a relative contraindication to initiation of testosterone therapy and Hct > 54% as an indication to stop therapy [14].

2.3.1 Risk of Thrombosis and Cardiovascular Disease in Testosterone-Induced Erythrocytosis

Erythrocytosis has been linked to arterial thrombosis, in the setting of polycythemia vera. However, there is no evidence of such linkage in secondary erythrocytosis such as testosterone-induced erythrocytosis or hypoxia-driven erythrocytosis. Meanwhile, the risk of cardiovascular disease has been found to be twofold greater in patients with high hematocrit groups [15]. Overall, the data have been variable with regard to the association of erythrocytosis to venous thromboembolism (VTE). A 5% increase in hematocrit has demonstrated increased VTE risk (HR: 1.46) [16]. In a retrospective cohort study of 8709 men with low serum testosterone concentrations (<300 ng/dL [10.4 nmol/L]) undergoing coronary angiography, men who were subsequently prescribed testosterone had a higher risk of a composite outcome of all-cause mortality, myocardial infarction (MI), and stroke than men who did not take testosterone (hazard ratio [HR] 1.29, 95% CI 1.04–1.58) [17]. The proposed mechanism relates to increased blood viscosity, slower clot formation kinetics, and reduced clot strength due to erythrocytosis which could result in mechanical interference of platelet and fibrin interaction with endothelium [18]. The graph in Fig. 2.1 shows the incremental relationship between whole blood viscosity and hematocrit level.

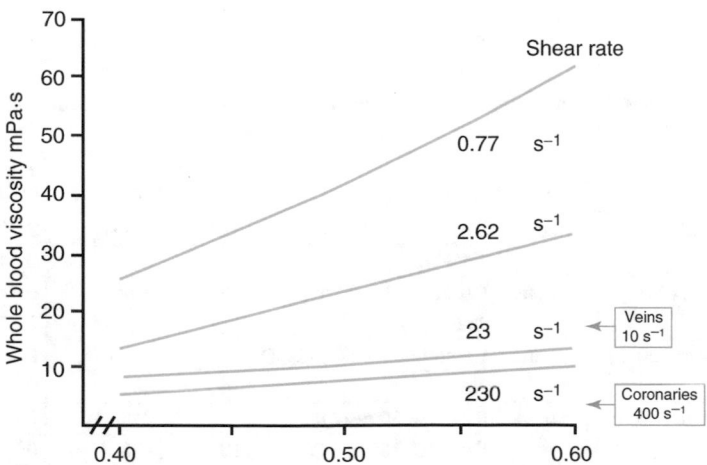

Fig. 2.1 Association between hematocrit level and whole blood viscosity. (The lines represent the relationship between the increase in whole blood viscosity levels and the increase in hematocrit levels among different levels of vasculature)

Studies have shown conflicting results pertaining to risk of VTE with testosterone-induced erythrocytosis. The Testosterone Trials study was a double-blind, placebo-controlled study which assigned 790 men of ages 65 years or older (with a serum testosterone concentration of less than 275 ng per deciliter and symptoms suggesting hypoandrogenism) to receive either testosterone gel or placebo gel for 1 year. The incidence of VTE was 1% among the 394 patients who received 1% testosterone gel, although it was not statistically significant compared to placebo [11]. Meanwhile, another multicenter, double-blind, randomized, placebo-controlled, 16-week trial with T solution 2% versus placebo conducted across medical centers in the United States, Canada, and Mexico showed no VTE occurrence among 36 patients receiving testosterone replacement [9]. Lastly, another study comparing the pharmacokinetics and treatment effectiveness of a topical testosterone gel (AA2500) found no incidence of VTE among the total of 317 participants who received testosterone gel [12].

The rates of thrombosis while on testosterone therapy in recent randomized trials are shown in Table 2.2. Overall, the prevalence of VTE ranged from 0% to 1.3% in the testosterone replacement groups.

Apart from the above randomized trials, two large population studies have been conducted to understand the association between testosterone therapy and VTE. The first trial studied 30,572 men >40 years of age and concluded that exposure to testosterone therapy in the last 15 days before the index event date was not associated with an increased risk of VTE (adjusted Odds Ratio (aOR), 0.90; 95% CI, 0.73–1.12) [19]. While the second study of 19,215 men showed that starting testosterone treatment was associated with increased risk of VTE (HR: 1.25), which peaked within 6 months and decreased thereafter as found among the men in the study [20]. Thus, the risk of VTE among patients with testosterone therapy remains an area of active investigation.

Table 2.2 Studies demonstrating the prevalence of erythrocytosis, cardiovascular disease, and venous thromboembolism in testosterone therapy

Study (year)	Time	Preparations	Sample size	Hct > 54%	MI/CVA	VTE
Snyder et al. (2016) [11]	2 years	T gel 1% 5 g QD initially	394	1.8%	2.3%	1%
		Placebo	394	0%	4.1%	1.3%
Brock et al. (2016) [8]	4 months	T solution 2% 60 mg QD	358	1.8%	0%	0%
		Placebo	357	0.3%	0.6%	0.6%
Paduch et al. (2015) [9]	4 months	T solution 2% 60 mg QD	36	0.8%	0%	0%
		Placebo	40	0%	0%	0%
Steidle et al. (2003) [12]	3 months	T gel 1% 50 mg QD	99	3%	0%	0%
		T gel 1% 100 mg QD	106	6%	0%	0%
		T patch 5 mg QD	102	1%	0%	0%
		Placebo	99	1%	0%	0%

Abbreviations: *T* testosterone, *QD* daily

2.3.2   Monitoring and Management of Erythrocytosis

The following clinical recommendations should be considered while prescribing testosterone therapy in patients. Transdermal or subcutaneous formulations should be strongly considered in at-risk populations in order to minimize significant alterations in hemoglobin and hematocrit values. For at-risk populations (type 2 diabetics, smokers, obese men), injectable testosterone formulations should be considered only after potential adverse hematological effects are discussed (Table 2.3). Additional risk factors like thrombophilia (e.g., factor V Leiden), antiphospholipid antibody syndrome (APLAS), prothrombin gene mutations, high factor VIII levels, and high homocysteine levels should be considered prior to starting testosterone therapy [21]. For patients who meet the criteria for and desire testosterone therapy, a baseline hemoglobin and hematocrit should be assessed. After initiation of therapy, the Sexual Medicine Society of North America advises that men should be "monitored regularly" for erythrocytosis [22]. Consensus International Society of Andrology (ISA), International Society for the Study of Aging Male (ISSAM), European Association of Urology (EAU), European Academy of Andrology, and American Society of Andrology guidelines advise that hemoglobin and hematocrit should be checked after 3–4 months, then after 1 year, and annually thereafter [23]. Based on the Endocrine Society Clinical Practice Guidelines, once Hct > 54% is reached, testosterone should either be discontinued or therapeutic phlebotomy be offered to reduce the risk of potential future thromboembolic events [14]. In the event of a thromboembolic episode for patients on testosterone therapy, we recommend discontinuing treatment and beginning anticoagulation per recommended guidelines [24]. More recently, there has been evidence to consider a diagnosis of obstructive sleep apnea (OSA) in hypogonadal men on testosterone replacement who develop secondary polycythemia [25].

The general management algorithm for patients in whom testosterone therapy is being considered is provided in Fig. 2.2.

Table 2.3 "At-risk" population for erythrocytosis	
	Hypoxia/cardiopulmonary-associated causes
	Smokers
	Obstructive sleep apnea/obesity hypoventilation syndrome
	Cyanotic heart disease
	Chronic pulmonary disease
	Kidney-associated causes
	History of renal transplant
	Renal artery stenosis
	Hematological causes
	Baseline borderline erythrocytosis

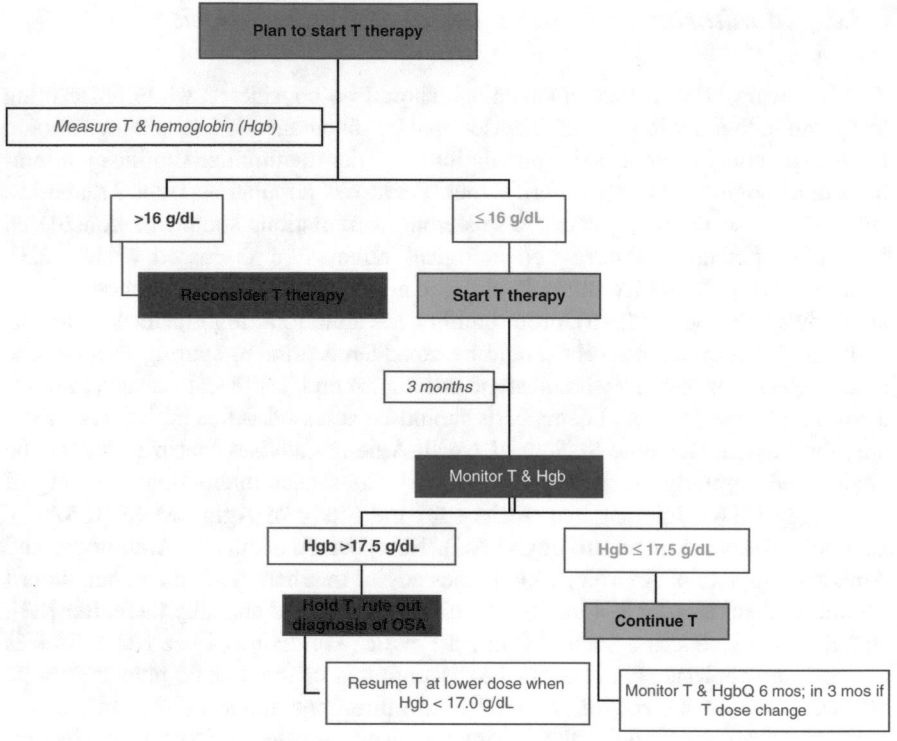

Fig. 2.2 Management of erythrocytosis on testosterone therapy

2.4 Conclusion

Erythrocytosis is uncommon while on testosterone therapy (<5%). However, monitoring is necessary to detect early erythrocytosis and minimize potential complications. The preponderance of randomized data suggest no increase in cardiovascular risk, while there currently is conflicting data on the risk of venous thromboembolism.

References

1. Baillargeon J, Urban RJ, Ottenbacher KJ, Pierson KS, Goodwin JS. Trends in androgen prescribing in the United States, 2001 to 2011. JAMA Intern Med. 2013;173(15):1465–6.
2. Corona G, Lee DM, Forti G, O'Connor DB, Maggi M, O'Neill TW, et al. Age-related changes in general and sexual health in middle-aged and older men: results from the European Male Ageing Study (EMAS). J Sex Med. 2010;7(4 pt 1):1362–80.
3. Mulligan T, Frick M, Zuraw Q, Stemhagen A, McWhirter C. Prevalence of hypogonadism in males aged at least 45 years: the HIM study. Int J Clin Pract. 2006;60(7):762–9.
4. Wu FC, Tajar A, Beynon JM, Pye SR, Silman AJ, Finn JD, et al. Identification of late-onset hypogonadism in middle-aged and elderly men. N Engl J Med. 2010;363(2):123–35.

5. Calof OM, Singh AB, Lee ML, Kenny AM, Urban RJ, Tenover JL, et al. Adverse events associated with testosterone replacement in middle-aged and older men: a meta-analysis of randomized, placebo-controlled trials. J Gerontol Ser A Biol Med Sci. 2005;60(11):1451–7.
6. Wintrobe MM. Wintrobe's clinical hematology. Lippincott Williams & Wilkins; 2008.
7. Hoffman R, Benz EJ Jr, Silberstein LE, Heslop H, Anastasi J, Weitz J. Hematology: basic principles and practice. Elsevier Health Sciences; 2013.
8. Brock G, Heiselman D, Maggi M, Kim SW, Rodríguez Vallejo JM, Behre HM, et al. Effect of testosterone solution 2% on testosterone concentration, sex drive and energy in hypogonadal men: results of a placebo controlled study. J Urol. 2016;195(3):699–705.
9. Paduch DA, Polzer PK, Ni X, Basaria S. Testosterone replacement in androgen-deficient men with ejaculatory dysfunction: a randomized controlled trial. J Clin Endocrinol Metabol. 2015;100(8):2956–62.
10. Ponce OJ, Spencer-Bonilla G, Alvarez-Villalobos N, Serrano V, Singh-Ospina N, Rodriguez-Gutierrez R, et al. The efficacy and adverse events of testosterone replacement therapy in hypogonadal men: a systematic review and meta-analysis of randomized, placebo-controlled trials. J Clin Endocrinol Metabol. 2018;103(5):1745–54.
11. Snyder PJ, Bhasin S, Cunningham GR, Matsumoto AM, Stephens-Shields AJ, Cauley JA, et al. Effects of testosterone treatment in older men. N Engl J Med. 2016;374(7):611–24.
12. Steidle C, Schwartz S, Jacoby K, Sebree T, Smith T, Bachand R, et al. AA2500 testosterone gel normalizes androgen levels in aging males with improvements in body composition and sexual function. J Clin Endocrinol Metabol. 2003;88(6):2673–81.
13. Bachman E, Feng R, Travison T, Li M, Olbina G, Ostland V, et al. Testosterone suppresses hepcidin in men: a potential mechanism for testosterone-induced erythrocytosis. J Clin Endocrinol Metabol. 2010;95(10):4743–7.
14. Bhasin S, Cunningham GR, Hayes FJ, Matsumoto AM, Snyder PJ, Swerdloff RS, et al. Testosterone therapy in men with androgen deficiency syndromes: an Endocrine Society clinical practice guideline. J Clin Endocrinol Metabol. 2010;95(6):2536–59.
15. Sorlie PD, Garcia-Palmieri MR, Costas R Jr, Havlik RJ. Hematocrit and risk of coronary heart disease: the Puerto Rico Heart Health Program. Am Heart J. 1981;101(4):456–61.
16. Brækkan SK, Mathiesen EB, Njølstad I, Wilsgaard T, Hansen J-B. Hematocrit and risk of venous thromboembolism in a general population. The Tromsø study. Haematologica. 2010;95(2):270–5.
17. Vigen R, O'Donnell CI, Barón AE, Grunwald GK, Maddox TM, Bradley SM, et al. Association of testosterone therapy with mortality, myocardial infarction, and stroke in men with low testosterone levels. JAMA. 2013;310(17):1829–36.
18. Shibata J, Hasegawa J, Siemens H-J, Wolber E, Dibbelt L, Li D, et al. Hemostasis and coagulation at a hematocrit level of 0.85: functional consequences of erythrocytosis. Blood. 2003;101(11):4416–22.
19. Baillargeon J, Urban RJ, Morgentaler A, Glueck CJ, Baillargeon G, Sharma G, et al., editors. Risk of venous thromboembolism in men receiving testosterone therapy. Mayo Clin Proc. 2015;90(8):1038–45. Elsevier.
20. Martinez C, Suissa S, Rietbrock S, Katholing A, Freedman B, Cohen AT, et al. Testosterone treatment and risk of venous thromboembolism: population based case-control study. BMJ. 2016;355:i5968.
21. Freedman J, Glueck CJ, Prince M, Riaz R, Wang P. Testosterone, thrombophilia, thrombosis. Transl Res. 2015;165(5):537–48.
22. Ohlander SJ, Varghese B, Pastuszak AW. Erythrocytosis following testosterone therapy. Sex Med Rev. 2018;6(1):77–85.
23. Wang C, Nieschlag E, Swerdloff R, Behre HM, Hellstrom WJ, Gooren LJ, et al. Investigation, treatment, and monitoring of late-onset hypogonadism in males: ISA, ISSAM, EAU, EAA, and ASA recommendations. J Androl. 2009;30(1):1–9.
24. Kearon C, Akl EA, Ornelas J, Blaivas A, Jimenez D, Bounameaux H, et al. Antithrombotic therapy for VTE disease: CHEST guideline and expert panel report. Chest. 2016;149(2):315–52.
25. Lundy SD, Parekh NV, Shoskes DA. Obstructive sleep apnea is associated with polycythemia in hypogonadal men on testosterone replacement therapy. J Sex Med. 2020;17(7):1297–303.

Chapter 3
Role of Gonadotropins in Adult-Onset Functional Hypogonadism

Ilpo Huhtaniemi

3.1 Introduction

The two main functions of the testis are the production of testosterone (T) and spermatogenesis. The endocrine regulation of these activities occurs along the hypothalamic-pituitary-testicular (HPT) axis (Fig. 3.1), where the key role is played by the two gonadotropic hormones produced by the anterior pituitary gland – luteinizing hormone (LH) and follicle-stimulating hormone (FSH) [23, 43]. The secretion of LH and FSH is stimulated by the hypothalamic gonadotropin-releasing hormone (GnRH), which is under negative feedback control via sex steroids [19]. GnRH neurons do not respond directly to androgen (T) and estrogen (estradiol) feedback, but mainly regulate GnRH release by inhibiting the production of kisspeptin, a proximal hypothalamic peptide hormone with stimulatory action on GnRH synthesis [42]. The negative feedback regulation of FSH additionally occurs at the level of the pituitary gland through action of the testicular peptide hormone inhibin B.

Balanced function (homeostasis) of the HPT axis, whereby gonadotropins maintain the physiological levels of testicular androgen production and spermatogenesis, and testicular hormones feed back to the hypothalamic-pituitary level to maintain the required gonadotropin stimulus, are the hallmark of male eugonadism. T deficiency, the pathognomonic finding in male hypogonadism, can occur at any age from the fetal period until old age. Hypogonadism can be *primary* or *hypergonadotropic (PH)*, when the testis tissue is unable to produce sufficient amounts of T and/or sperm despite sufficient gonadotropin simulation. In this case, the lack of gonadal negative feedback brings about elevated gonadotropin levels. The other form of hypogonadism, termed *secondary* or *hypogonadotropic (SH)*, is caused by low or inappropriately normal (i.e., insufficient) gonadotropin secretion that is unable to

I. Huhtaniemi (✉)
Institute of Reproductive and Developmental Biology, Department of Metabolism, Digestion and Reproduction, Imperial College London, London, UK
e-mail: ilpo.huhtaniemi@imperial.ac.uk

© Springer Nature Switzerland AG 2021
J. P. Mulhall et al. (eds.), *Controversies in Testosterone Deficiency*,
https://doi.org/10.1007/978-3-030-77111-9_3

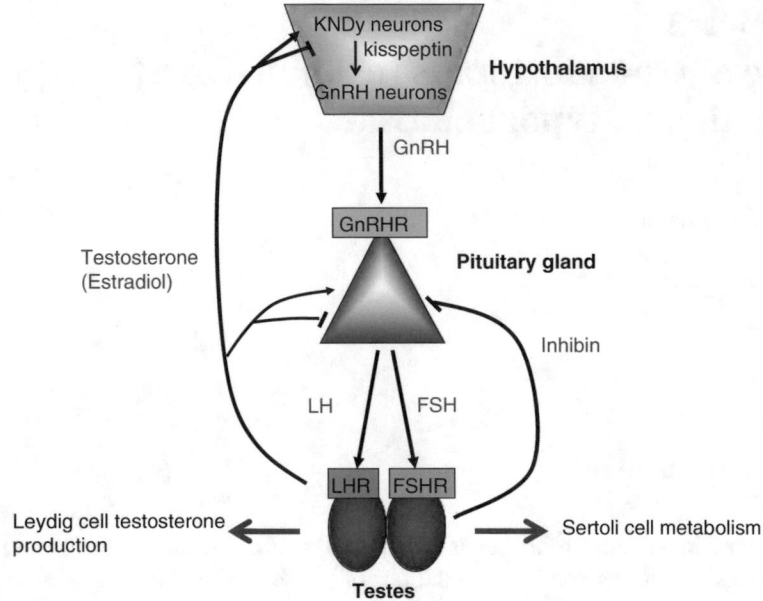

Fig. 3.1 The hypothalamic-pituitary-testicular axis. Abbreviations: KNDy, kisspeptin, neurokinin B, dynorphin; GnRH, gonadotropin-releasing hormone; R, receptor; LH, luteinizing hormone; FSH, follicle-stimulating hormone

support testicular function. It can be caused by deficiency of the pituitary gonadotrope cells to produce gonadotropins or by the lack of their hypothalamic stimulation by GnRH and/or kisspeptin. Gonadotropin measurements therefore form an essential part in the differential diagnosis between PH and SH.

Another way to classify hypogonadism is to divide it into *organic (OH)* and *functional (FH)* hypogondism. OH is the classical form of hypogonadism caused by a structural, functional, or genetic disturbance at one of the levels of the HPT axis, often congenital and usually irreversible. FH, also historically termed late-onset hypogonadism (LOH) or andropause, occurs usually in adulthood and is often associated with comorbidities and/or old age. LOH can be considered a misnomer because comorbidities (in particular obesity) are more important causes for the condition than advanced age. As a general rule, T levels in FH are not as profoundly reduced as they are in OH, and they may be reversible. Also, FH can be primary or secondary, but often the patient has mixed features of both. In cases of secondary FH, the etiology is more often a comorbidity (e.g., obesity), while OH is more commonly due to primary hypothalamic or testicular dysgenesis issues. Purely age-dependent hypogonadism is likely less common and typically is due to primary testicular insufficiency [55]. Compensated or subclinical hypogonadism (CH), wherein gonadotropin levels are elevated in the setting of normal T, is less well defined and may occur with either OH or FH and may represent a precursor condition of hypogonadism in some cases [12, 45].

The purpose of this review is to discuss the role of gonadotropins in the pathogenesis, diagnosis, and treatment of different types of male FH.

3.2 Gonadotropin Measurements

3.2.1 Gonadotropin Assays

The sandwich-type immunometric methods currently used in clinical laboratories have high specificity and sensitivity (down to 0.05–0.1 IU/L) for LH and FSH, allowing reliable detection of the concentrations of male patients in most physiological and pathophysiological situations [53]. The reference range for LH in adult men is commonly reported between 1.5 and 8.5 IU/L, while FSH is reported to be 1.5–12.5 IU/L. However, in the setting of infertility, lower thresholds have been reported to indicate subfertility, including maximal FSH levels of 4.6–7.6 IU/L. Individual results should be interpreted against a reference range established by regional laboratories in healthy men from a representative local general population. Due to the pulsatile secretion and short half-life (20 min) of circulating LH, multiple measurements, or pooling of 2–3 individual samples, can be used to reduce sample-to-sample variability. In contrast, the half-life of FSH is longer (3–4 h), and a single measurement of this hormone is usually sufficient.

Gonadotropin assays used today in clinical laboratories are reliable with rare technical problems. Heterophilic antibodies in patient serum can be a rare cause of erroneously high gonadotropin levels [54]. There is a common genetic polymorphism of the *LHB* gene (W8R/I15T), with 10–20% allelic frequency in various populations, giving rise to an immunological variant of LH that is not detected by some immunometric assays, especially those using antibodies against the LH α/β dimer [29]. An inappropriately low level of LH is found in carriers of the polymorphic gene, even though the bioactivity of the aberrant hormone is roughly normal. Such an unexpected finding should be verified by another assay using a different combination of antibodies. Inactivating mutations of gonadotropin subunit genes and inactivating and activating mutation of gonadotropin receptor genes are extremely rare causes of inappropriate gonadotropin levels, unlikely to be found in men with FH.

3.2.2 Gonadotropin Bioactivity, Polymorphisms, and Microheterogeneity

Older studies have reported that low gonadotropin levels (such as in hypogonadotropic hypogonadism) have a low ratio of bioactivity to immunoreactivity, as measured by in vitro bioassay and competitive immunoassay [44, 49]. It has more recently been established that such apparent bioimmuno ratio differences were due to overestimation of low concentrations by older immunoassays [22, 27]. The understanding now is that the quality of gonadotropins throughout the concentration range occurring in men does not change, suggesting that the current immunometric methods are functionally relevant. Admittedly, circulating gonadotropins display microheterogeneity due to variations in the degree of glycosylation of individual molecules [4], but the clinical relevance of this phenomenon is likely marginal.

There are several common polymorphisms in gonadotropin subunit and receptor genes [7, 29, 37], which have been shown to influence the basal circulating levels of gonadotropins. Determination of the polymorphisms may, therefore, help identify one reason for an unexpected gonadotropin finding in hypogonadism. Alternatively, a GnRH stimulation test may be performed to evaluate responsiveness of the HPT axis [2].

3.2.3 Interpretation of the Findings

The first suspicion of hypogonadism is based on symptoms (and signs) and low concentration of peripheral serum T. Due to significant day-to-day and diurnal variability in T levels, at least two tests should be obtained from fasting blood samples within several hours of waking. If T levels are low, basal gonadotropin secretion should be measured in the peripheral serum to differentiate between PH and SH. Defining PH vs SH is clinically important, as it provides prognostic information (i.e., reversible vs non-reversible), may lead to further diagnostic testing (i.e., prolactin, pituitary MRI), and influences treatment options. In cases where fertility is not relevant, LH measurement is usually sufficient without the need for FSH. However, as FSH and LH are typically concordant, FSH may be ordered in cases where the diagnosis of PH vs SH is unclear to provide further information about pituitary activity.

Occasionally, GnRH stimulation testing may be useful to clarify indeterminate findings, such as in men with normal LH and low T [2]. Following GnRH stimulation, a low gonadotropin response suggests malfunction at the pituitary level, whereas increases in gonadotropins and testosterone suggest impairment at the hypothalamic level. Similarly, human chorionic gonadotropin (hCG) stimulation can be used to assess the testicular steroidogenic capacity when primary hypogonadism is suspected [2, 13]. Bang et al. [2] recently reported reference ranges for gonadotropin and T responses following GnRH and hGG stimulation tests in healthy men as well as in men with various forms of hypogonadism. Results obtained in obese men with suspected FH demonstrated normal LH responses to GnRH stimulation, suggesting that the low basal gonadotropin levels were more commonly secondary to inadequate hormonal release at the hypothalamic level [46]. A similar finding of maintained pituitary responsiveness to GnRH has been reported in aging men [39]. In contrast, hCG stimulation in obese men resulted in diminished T response at the level of the testicle [2, 26, 40], possibly due to the negative influence of adipose tissue-derived hormones on Leydig cell function. Interestingly, common polymorphisms of gonadotropin subunit and receptor genes have marginal effects on gonadotropin concentrations and receptor activity, and thus do not influence the results of GnRH or hCG stimulation tests [2].

3.3   Pathogenesis of Functional Hypogonadism (FH)

FH has been used to describe a milder form of hypogonadism which results from chronic disease, stress, inadequate nutrition, obesity, and/or old age [17]. Unlike OH, FH can often be transient and/or reversible, depending on the nature of the etiology. FH should only be diagnosed after exclusion of OH and should not be assumed based on age alone. For example, Klinefelter syndrome represents a common etiology for OH but may not be diagnosed until later in life [16].

FH can, in principle, occur at any age, although it may occur more commonly in older men. In both children and adults, it may be caused by multiple systemic diseases (see [3, 57]), with obesity, arguably, representing the most common etiology. Although most studies have focused on low T in men with obesity, lesser attention has been directed to the other part of testicular function, spermatogenesis. As will be discussed below, suppressed spermatogenesis may also occur in a distinct subgroup of men with FH. This condition may often go unnoticed in older men, as fertility is often a lesser concern in this population.

Because of differing etiologies, clinical management and prognosis of primary and secondary FH are often different. It is helpful to differentiate men into different diagnostic categories according to their T and gonadotropin levels. Based on results from 3119 community-dwelling men aged 40–79 years (EMAS study) [45], four distinct categories were defined (Fig. 3.2): (1) normal T and LH (eugonadism – 76.7%), (2) low T and high LH (PH – 2.0%), (3) low T and low-to-normal LH (SH – 11.8%), and (4) normal T and high LH (CH – 9.5%). It is noteworthy that when the definition for hypogonadism included both abnormal levels and symptoms (i.e., sexual symptoms), the rates of hypogonadism declined significantly. It is important to emphasize the need of gonadotropin measurements to define the diagnosis (see also below), because, at least in the United States, only 12% of men with FH have their LH and/or FSH measured before the initiation of T replacement therapy [33]. The distinction may also help contribute to the selection of therapy for men, particularly among those desiring to maintain fertility.

3.3.1   Primary (Hypergonadotropic) Hypogonadism

Primary hypogonadism is diagnosed through both low T and usually elevated LH. In most cases, FSH is more elevated than LH, and as such, it may be used as an adjunctive test in cases where the diagnosis is in question [32]. Although PH is a common etiology among the classical early-onset hypogonadism (OH), it may also occur in older men, particularly among those with comorbid conditions [56].

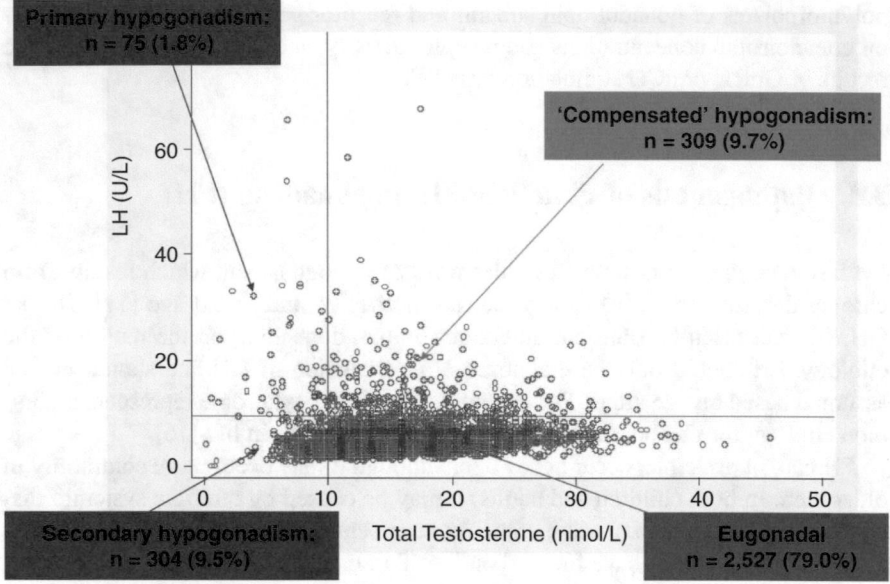

Fig. 3.2 Correlation of testosterone and LH levels in the EMAS population [45], a cohort of 3016 community-dwelling men in aged 40–79 years in eight European centers (UK, Sweden, Belgium, Estonia, Poland, Hungary, Italy, and Spain). The *vertical line* corresponds to lower limit of normal total T (10.5 nmol/l) and the *horizontal line* corresponds to upper limit of normal LH (9.4 U/l). The population can be divided into eugonadal (T > 10.5 nmol/L; LH > 9.4 IU/L); primary hypogonadal (T < 10.5 nmol/L; LH > 9.4 IU/L), secondary hypogonadal (T < 10.5 nmol/L; LH > 9.4 IU/L), and men with compensatory hypogonadism (T > 10.5 nmol/L; LH > 9.4 IU/L). (Modified from Tajar et al. [45])

In some cases of PH, a man may have normal T and LH but elevated FSH. This situation may occur following radio- or chemotherapy, where spermatogenesis but not steroidogenesis may be impaired, while in other cases, it may be idiopathic [15].

Multiple mechanisms are associated with elevated LH in aging independent of comorbid states. They include age-related decreases of Leydig cell mass [34], testicular blood perfusion [41], and biochemical function [50], which are further exacerbated in conditions of poor health. Impaired testicular response to LH can also be caused by elevated cytokine levels [20, 48] associated with low-grade inflammation common in aging [18]. Primary testicular failure can also occur in connection with alcohol abuse [8], renal disease [25], COPD [28], and malignancy [14].

3.3.2 Secondary (Hypogonadotropic) Hypogonadism

It is important to identify men with SH, because it may be caused by significant pathologies, including pituitary or hypothalamic tumors, panhypopituitarism, or be due to acute illness, medications (e.g., glucocorticoids or opioids), or obesity.

Secondary hypogonadism is often reversible through treating comorbidities, changing offending medications, and optimizing lifestyle factors [6].

Obesity-related suppression of HPT function has several possible mechanisms, including the pleiotropic inhibitory effects of adipocyte-produced adipokines, cytokines, and chemokines on GnRH and gonadotropin secretion [47], as well as obesity-related central insulin resistance [5, 36], which may negate the stimulatory effect of insulin on gonadotropin secretion. One candidate peptide associated with obesity-related HPT suppression is the fat-cell-produced leptin, which is reduced in men receiving T therapy [30, 31]. Additionally, proinflammatory fat tissue cytokines (e.g., tumor necrosis factor, IL-2, and IL-6) may further suppress gonadotropin secretion [51]. Other substances have shown similar suppressive effects, including endocannabinoids [35] and adiponectin [9]. Finally, lower SHBG in obesity may lower the set point of HPT feedback inhibition. As total T is predominantly suppressed in obesity, free T remains relatively higher and able to inhibit gonadotropins at lower levels of circulating total T. Interestingly, the long-held hypothesis that increases in adipose tissue result in reduced T levels due to increased estradiol feedback has been challenged by more recent findings [45].

3.3.3 Mixed Primary/Secondary Hypogonadism

The combination of both PH and SH is relatively common, especially among aged obese men, where the primary age-dependent derangement of testicular tissues and comorbidity-associated suppression of HPT function overlap. Similarly, adipokines produced by fat tissue have inhibitory effects on both hypothalamic GnRH secretion on Leydig cell steroidogenesis [40].

3.3.4 Compensated Hypogonadism

Elevated gonadotropins with normal T (LH >9.4 IU/L; T ≥ 10.5 nmol/L) is a common finding in aging men, representing 9.5% in the previously described EMAS cohort overall (Fig. 3.2) and 21% of men aged 70–79 [45]. A different cohort of >4000 men presenting to a sexual dysfunction clinic reported a lower prevalence rate of CH (4.1%), which likely relates to differences in study populations and suggests that men with CH are less likely to potentially exhibit low T-related symptoms [11]. Given these observations, the clinical significance of the isolated LH elevation is unclear. However, several clinically relevant issues related to CH include identifying associated or underlying etiologies and documenting hypogonadal symptoms. Additionally, further research is warranted to determine if CH is able to predict future health conditions, including uncompensated hypogonadism.

Although the exact cause of isolated LH elevation in these men is unknown, it may relate to T suppression that has occurred within the defined "normal" reference range and therefore goes essentially unnoticed. With this hypothesis, these men would normally have T levels in the mid to upper eugonadal range (e.g., 30 nmol/L), and even with 70% suppression (11 nmol/L), they would still be considered normal. In cases such as this, hypogonadal symptoms may be more likely to occur in CH. Interestingly, in the EMAS cohort, men with CH had no sexual symptoms after adjustment for age, BMI, smoking status, alcohol intake, and comorbidity [45]. However, their inability to do vigorous activity after adjustments persisted. This may suggest mild T deficiency, since when the T thresholds of the different hypogonadal symptoms were compared, the thresholds of suppressed physical activity were reported at 13 nmol/L, while those of various sexual domains ranged between 8 and 11 nmol/L [55]. Hence, although many men with CH are not overtly hypogondal, they may exhibit borderline symptoms of T deficiency. Whether they truly exhibit high baseline T levels when eugonadal remains an unproven hypothesis.

CH may also represent an intermediary stage in the transition from eugonadism to PH. When the testicular capacity to produce T starts waning as a result of various factors, the negative feedback of T on gonadotropin secretion decreases and serum LH increases. Initially, elevations in LH are able to maintain normal T levels (CH). When testicular function deteriorates further, the pituitary is unable to further compensate and PH ensues. As the latter is commonly associated with chronological aging [56], we would similarly expect aging to be associated with CH. In reviewing findings from EMAS, this finding was indeed observed, with the overall cohort having a mean age of 58.5, CH of 67.3, and PH of 70.0 [45].

The suggestion of CH being a harbinger of impending PH was also supported by findings from the 4.3-year prospective data obtained during the EMAS study [12]. In the study cohort, 5.2% of the men experienced incident CH (i.e., developed CH during the follow-up period), while 6.6% had persistent CH and 2.4% reverted to eugonadism during follow-up. Men with CH at baseline, indeed, had a 15-fold higher risk to subsequently develop PH at follow-up than men with baseline normal LH and T [12]. The development of CH was associated with several factors, including age > 70 years, diabetes, chronic pain, pre-degree education, and low physical activity. These men also developed erectile dysfunction, poor health, CVD, and cancer more frequently, and their cognitive and physical function deteriorated more than in men with persistently normal LH.

Other supporting findings of the concept of CH include lower hemoglobin levels, erectile dysfunction, poor health, cardiovascular disease, cognitive and physical deterioration, and cancer compared to eugonadal men [12]. It could therefore be concluded that elevated LH in the presence of normal T is not an incidental finding. Although it may revert to normal levels spontaneously, it remains associated with multiple signs and symptoms of deteriorating health. However, at the present time, isolated elevations in LH are not an unequivocal biomarker of hypogonadism.

Several other studies support the finding that elevated LH in the setting of normal T may be associated with other medical conditions. Hyde and colleagues reported that increased LH was a risk factor for ischemic heart disease in older men [24]. The same conclusion was made by another study on CH where elevated LH was associated with psychiatric and cardiovascular symptoms, but not specifically with sexual symptoms [11]. These men were also more likely to develop PH compared to men with normal LH and T. A study from Denmark [21] found a positive association with elevated LH but not T and all-cause mortality, suggesting that CH may be a risk factor for early death. These preliminary findings underpin the potential clinical importance of detecting CH in the diagnostic work-up of men with suspected hypogonadism.

Another cohort study by Ventimiglia et al. [52] provided additional and somewhat contrasting information on CH in relation to other forms of hypogonadism. In their analysis of infertile, hypogonadal men, the authors stratified groups into PH, SH, and CH according to the EMAS criteria [45]. Results showed that CH represented a mild form of PH, while no differences in age were noted between groupings. Similar to the EMAS study, obesity was common among all men, with SH displaying the highest overall risk. Testicular volume was low, FSH high, and inhibin B low in both CH and PH. Impaired spermatogenesis was also identified in men with CH, which is not commonly evaluated in aging male studies.

3.4 Gonadotropins in the Treatment of Functional Hypogonadism

The first line of treatment for FH is lifestyle modifications, including weight reduction, dietary optimization, medication review, and treatment of comorbidities, after which T therapy can be considered in men with no contraindications [10]. If maintained fertility is desired, exogenous T is contraindicated, except in certain scenarios, as it reduces gonadotropins and intratesticular T below the threshold required to maintain spermatogenesis. In this setting, gonadotropin treatment may be useful in men with SH but not PH. One meta-analysis of men with organic SH reported outcomes of men who received gonadotropins and demonstrated successful results (mean sperm count 6 mil/mL and with at least one spermatozoon in ejaculate) in 75% of patients [38]. Improved success rates were noted among men who received both human chorionic gonadotropin (hCG) and FSH compared to hCG alone. Similar beneficial results were also observed among men who receive GnRH therapy.

Other fertility-preserving alternatives to treat hypogonadism include aromatase inhibitors (e.g., letrozole and anastrozole) or selective estrogen receptor modulators (SERMs; e.g., clomiphene citrate and enclomiphene citrate), both of which increase gonadotropin levels by reducing the negative feedback at the hypothalamic level, thus potentiating the stimulation of intratesticular T and spermatogenesis. Aromatase inhibitors are generally not recommended for extended use because of their variable efficacy and deleterious effects on bone mineral density. SERMs might be a better alternative to achieve the same goal; however, more research is required to better evaluate their efficacy and long-term safety profile [1].

References

1. Awouters M, Vanderschueren D, Antonio L. Aromatase inhibitors and selective estrogen receptor modulators: unconventional therapies for functional hypogonadism? Andrology. 2019. https://doi.org/10.1111/andr.12725.
2. Bang AK, Nordkap L, Almstrup K, Priskorn L, Petersen JH, Rajpert-De Meyts E, et al. Dynamic GnRH and hCG testing: establishment of new diagnostic reference levels. Eur J Endocrinol. 2017;176:379–91.
3. Boehm U, Bouloux PM, Dattani MT, de Roux N, Dodé C, Dunkel L, et al. Expert consensus document: European Consensus Statement on congenital hypogonadotropic hypogonadism – pathogenesis, diagnosis and treatment. Nat Rev Endocrinol. 2015;11:547–64.
4. Bousfield GR, Dias JA. Synthesis and secretion of gonadotropins including structure-function correlates. Rev Endocr Metab Disord. 2011;12:289–302.
5. Brüning JC, Gautam D, Burks DJ, Gillette J, Schubert M, Orban PC, et al. Role of brain insulin receptor in control on body weight and reproduction. Science. 2000;289:2122–5.
6. Camacho EM, Huhtaniemi IT, O'Neill TW, Finn JD, Pye SR, et al. Age-associated changes in hypothalamic–pituitary– testicular function in middle-aged and older men are modified by weight change and lifestyle factors: longitudinal results from the European male ageing study. Eur J Endocrinol. 2013;168:445–55.
7. Casarini L, Pignatti E, Simoni M. Effects of polymorphisms in gonadotropin and gonadotropin receptor genes on reproductive function. Rev Endocr Metab Disord. 2011;12:303–21.
8. Castilla-García A, Santolaria-Fernández FJ, González-Reimers CE, Batista-López N, González-García C, Jorge-Hernández JA, Hernández-Nieto L. Alcohol induced hypogonadism: reversal after ethanol withdrawal. Drug Alcohol Depend. 1987;20:255–60.
9. Cheng XB, Wen JP, Yang J, Yang Y, Ning G, Li XY. GnRH secretion is inhibited by adiponectin through activation of AMP-activated protein kinase and extracellular signal-regulated kinase. Endocrine. 2011;39:6–12.
10. Corona G, Goulis DG, Huhtaniemi I, Zitzmann M, Toppari J, Forti G, et al. European Academy of Andrology (EAA) guidelines on investigation, treatment and monitoring of functional hypogonadism in males. Andrology. 2020. https://doi.org/10.1111/andr.12770.
11. Corona G, Maseroli E, Rastrelli G, Sforza A, Forti G, Mannucci E, et al. Characteristics of compensated hypogonadism in patients with sexual dysfunction. J Sex Med. 2014;11:1823–34.
12. Eendebak RJAH, Ahern T, Swiecicka A, Pye SR, O'Neill TW, Bartfai G, et al. Elevated luteinizing hormone despite normal testosterone levels in older men-natural history, risk factors and clinical features. Clin Endocrinol. 2018;88:479–90.
13. Forest MG. How should we perform the human chorionic gonadotrophin (hCG) stimulation test? Int J Androl. 1983;6:1–4.
14. Garcia JM, Li H, Mann D, Epner D, Hayes TG, Marcelli M, Cunningham GR. Hypogonadism in male patients with cancer. Cancer. 2006;106:2583–91.
15. Giannetta E, Gianfrilli D, Barbagallo F, Isidori AM, Lenzi A. Subclinical male hypogonadism. Best Pract Res Clin Endocrinol Metab. 2010;26:539–50.
16. Gravholt CH, Chang S, Wallentin M, Fedder J, Moore P, Skakkebæk A. Klinefelter syndrome: integrating genetics, neuropsychology, and endocrinology. Endocr Rev. 2018;39:389–423.
17. Grossmann M, Matsumoto AM. A perspective on middle-aged and older men with functional hypogonadism: focus on holistic management. J Clin Endocrinol Metab. 2017;102:1067–75.
18. Haring R, Baumeister SE, Völzke H, Dörr M, Kocher T, Nauck M, et al. Prospective inverse associations of sex hormone concentrations in men with biomarkers of inflammation and oxidative stress. J Androl. 2012;33:944–50.
19. Herbison AE. Physiology of the adult gonadotropin-releasing hormone neuronal network. In: Plant TM, Zeleznik AJ, editors. Knobil and Neil's physiology of reproduction, vol. 1. 4th ed. Waltham: Academic Press; 2015. p. 399–467.

20. Hong CY, Park JH, Ahn RS, Im SY, Choi HS, Soh J, et al. Molecular mechanism of suppression of testicular steroidogenesis by proinflammatory cytokine tumor necrosis factor alpha. Mol Cell Biol. 2004;24:2593–604.
21. Holmboe SA, Vradi E, Kold Jensen T, Linneberg A, Husemoen LLN, Scheike T, et al. The association of reproductive hormone levels and all-cause, cancer, and cardiovascular disease mortality in men. J Clin Endocrinol Metab. 2015;100:4472–80.
22. Huhtaniemi I, Ding YQ, Tähtelä R, Välimäki M. The bio/immuno ratio of plasma luteinizing hormone does not change during the endogenous secretion pulse: reanalysis of the concept using improved immunometric techniques. J Clin Endocrinol Metab. 1992;75(6):1442–5.
23. Huhtaniemi IT, Howard S, Dunkel L, Anderson RA. The gonadal axis: a life perspective. In: Pfaff DW, Joels M, editors. Hormones, brain, and behavior. 3rd ed. London: Elsevier; 2017. p. 3–58.
24. Hyde Z, Norman PE, Flicker L, et al. Elevated LH predicts ischaemic heart disease events in older men: the Health in Men Study. Eur J Endocrinol. 2011;164:569–77.
25. Iglesias P, Carrero JJ, Díez JJ. Gonadal dysfunction in men with chronic kidney disease: clinical features, prognostic implications and therapeutic options. J Nephrol. 2012;25:31–42.
26. Isidori AM, Caprio M, Strollo F, Moretti C, Frajese G, Isidori A, et al. Leptin and androgens in male obesity: evidence for leptin contribution to reduced androgen levels. J Clin Endocrinol Metab. 1999;84:3673–80.
27. Jaakkola T, Ding YQ, Kellokumpu-Lehtinen P, Valavaara R, Martikainen H, Tapanainen J, et al. The ratios of serum bioactive/immunoreactive luteinizing hormone and follicle-stimulating hormone in various clinical conditions with increased and decreased gonadotropin secretion: reevaluation by a highly sensitive immunometric assay. J Clin Endocrinol Metab. 1990;70:1496–505.
28. Kamischke A, Kemper DE, Castel MA, Lüthke M, Rolf C, Behre HM, et al. Testosterone levels in men with chronic obstructive pulmonary disease with or without glucocorticoid therapy. Eur Respir J. 1998;11:41–5.
29. Lamminen T, Huhtaniemi I. A common genetic variant of luteinizing hormone; relation to normal and aberrant pituitary-gonadal function. Eur J Pharmacol. 2001;414:1–7.
30. Landry D, Cloutier F, Martin LJ. Implications of leptin in neuroendocrine regulation of male reproduction. Reprod Biol. 2013;13:1–14.
31. Luukkaa V, Pesonen U, Huhtaniemi I, Lehtonen A, Tilvis R, Tuomilehto J, Koulu M, Huupponen R. Inverse correlation between serum testosterone and leptin in men. J Clin Endocrinol Metab. 1998;83:3243–6.
32. Morley JE, Kaiser FE, Perry HM 3rd, Patrick P, Morley PM, Stauber PM, et al. Longitudinal changes in testosterone, luteinizing hormone, and follicle-stimulating hormone in healthy older men. Metabolism. 1997;46:410–3.
33. Muram D, Zhang X, Cui Z, Matsumoto AM. Use of hormone testing for the diagnosis and evaluation of male hypogonadism and monitoring of testosterone therapy: application of hormone testing guideline recommendations in clinical practice. J Sex Med. 2015;12:1886–94.
34. Neaves WB, Johnson L, Porter JC, Parker CR Jr, Petty CS. Leydig cell numbers, daily sperm production, and serum gonadotropin levels in aging men. J Clin Endocrinol Metab. 1984;59:756–63.
35. Pagotto U, Marsicano G, Cota D, Lutz B, Pasquali R. The emerging role of the endocannabinoid system in endocrine regulation and energy balance. Endocr Rev. 2006;27:73–100.
36. Porte D Jr, Baskin DG, Schwartz MW. Insulin signaling in the central nervous system: a critical role in metabolic homeostasis and disease from C. elegans to humans. Diabetes. 2005;54:1264–76.
37. Punab AM, Grigorova M, Punab M, Adler M, Kuura T, Poolamets O, et al. Carriers of variant luteinizing hormone (V-LH) among 1593 Baltic men have significantly higher serum LH. Andrology. 2015;3:512–9.
38. Rastrelli G, Corona G, Mannucci E, Maggi M. Factors affecting spermatogenesis upon gonadotropin-replacement therapy: a meta-analytic study. Andrology. 2014;2:794–808.

39. Roelfsema F, Liu PY, Takahashi PY, Yang RJ, Veldhuis JD. Dynamic interactions between LH and testosterone in healthy community-dwelling men: impact of age and body composition. J Clin Endocrinol Metab. 2020;105:1–14.
40. Roumaud P, Martin LJ. Roles of leptin, adiponectin and resistin in the transcriptional regulation of steroidogenic genes contributing to decreased Leydig cells function in obesity. Horm Mol Biol Clin Investig. 2015;24:25–45.
41. Sasano N, Ichijo S. Vascular patterns of the human testis with special reference to its senile changes. Tohoku J Exp Med. 1969;99:269–80.
42. Skorupskaite K, George JT, Anderson RA. The kisspeptin-GnRH pathway in human reproductive health and disease. Hum Reprod Update. 2014;20:485–500.
43. Smith LB, Walker WH. Hormone signaling in the testis. In: Plant TM, Zeleznik AJ, editors. Knobil and Neil's physiology of reproduction, vol. 1. 4th ed. Waltham: Academic Press; 2015. p. 637–90.
44. St-Arnaud R, Lachance R, Kelly SJ, Belanger A, Dupont A, Labrie F. Loss of luteinizing hormone bioactivity in patients with prostatic cancer treated with an LHRH agonist and a pure antiandrogen. Clin Endocrinol. 1986;24:21–30.
45. Tajar A, Forti G, O'Neill TW, Lee DM, Silman AJ, Finn JD, et al. Characteristics of secondary, primary, and compensated hypogonadism in aging men: evidence from the European Male Ageing Study. J Clin Endocrinol Metab. 2010;95:1810–8.
46. Tripathy D, Dhindsa S, Garg R, Khaishagi A, Syed T, Dandona P. Hypogonadotropic hypogonadism in erectile dysfunction associated with type 2 diabetes mellitus: a common defect? Metab Syndr Relat Disord. 2003;1:75–80.
47. Tsatsanis C, Dermitzaki E, Avgoustinaki P, Malliaraki N, Mytaras V, Margioris AN. The impact of adipose tissue-derived factors on the hypothalamic-pituitary-gonadal (HPG) axis. Hormones (Athens). 2015;14:549–62.
48. van der Poll T, Romijn JA, Endert E, Sauerwein HP. Effects of tumor necrosis factor on the hypothalamic-pituitary-testicular axis in healthy men. Metabolism. 1993;42:303–7.
49. Veldhuis JD, Dufau ML. Estradiol modulates the pulsatile secretion of biologically active luteinizing hormone in man. J Clin Invest. 1987;80:631–8.
50. Veldhuis JD, Liu PY, Keenan DM, Takahashi PY. Older men exhibit reduced efficacy of and heightened potency downregulation by intravenous pulses of recombinant human LH: a study in 92 healthy men. Am J Physiol Endocrinol Metab. 2012;302:E117–22.
51. Veldhuis J, Yang R, Roelfsema F, Takahashi P. Proinflammatory cytokine infusion attenuates LH's feedforward on testosterone secretion: modulation by age. J Clin Endocrinol Metab. 2016;101:539–49.
52. Ventimiglia E, Ippolito S, Capogrosso P, Pederzoli F, Cazzaniga W, Boeri L, et al. Primary, secondary and compensated hypogonadism: a novel risk stratification for infertile men. Andrology. 2017;5:505–10.
53. Wheeler MJ. Assays for LH, FSH, and prolactin. Methods Mol Biol. 2006;324:109–24.
54. Witherspoon LR, Witkin M, Shuler SE, Neely H, Gilbert S. Heterophilic antibody as source of error in immunoassay. South Med J. 1986;79:836–9.
55. Wu FC, Tajar A, Beynon JM, Pye SR, Silman AJ, Finn JD, et al. Identification of late-onset hypogonadism in middle-aged and elderly men. N Engl J Med. 2010;363:123–35.
56. Wu FC, Tajar A, Pye SR, Silman AJ, Finn JD, O'Neill TW, et al. Hypothalamic-pituitary-testicular axis disruptions in older men are differentially linked to age and modifiable risk factors: the European Male Aging Study. J Clin Endocrinol Metab. 2008;93:2737–45.
57. Young J, Xu C, Papadakis GE, Acierno JS, Maione L, Hietamäki J, Raivio T, et al. Clinical management of congenital hypogonadotropic hypogonadism. Endocr Rev. 2019;40:669–710.

Chapter 4
Hyperprolactinemia in Men with Testosterone Deficiency

Landon Trost

4.1 Introduction

The appropriate diagnosis and management of male testosterone (T) deficiency requires a thorough understanding of several physiologic processes and may require the integration of subspecialty services. The lack of understanding or appreciation of the complex nuances of low T may lead to missed diagnoses, inappropriate therapy, and potentially significant ramifications to a patient's overall health and well-being. One of these nuances includes the role and relevance of prolactin (PRL) and, more specifically, hyperprolactinemia as an important clinical condition. However, despite its importance, relatively few clinicians who treat low T have significant experience in managing PRL abnormalities. Given this observation, the objective of this chapter is to provide the practicing clinician a practical guide to evaluating and managing hyperprolactinemia. To accomplish this objective, the chapter is outlined to review the anatomy and physiology of PRL, associated findings and symptoms, its causative role in low T, the appropriate evaluation of hyperprolactinemia, and available management strategies. Although many clinicians may simply choose to refer men with hyperprolactinemia to an endocrinologist, a deeper understanding of these principles remains relevant, given that the initial diagnosis of hyperprolactinemia is most often dependent upon the sexual medicine clinician.

L. Trost (✉)
Male Fertility and Peyronie's Clinic, Orem, UT, USA
e-mail: email@mfp.clinic

© Springer Nature Switzerland AG 2021
J. P. Mulhall et al. (eds.), *Controversies in Testosterone Deficiency*,
https://doi.org/10.1007/978-3-030-77111-9_4

4.2   Prolactin and Hypothalamic-Pituitary-Gonadal Axis

Prolactin is a hormone produced in the anterior pituitary gland that serves predominantly to facilitate milk production in women. Several different actions lead to PRL secretion, including nursing, estrogen therapy/hormones, sexual activity, eating, and ovulation. As with other pituitary hormones, PRL is secreted in a pulsatile fashion and often occurs between stimulating events. It has additionally been suggested to have roles in immunomodulation and cell growth and differentiation and is particularly involved in hematopoiesis and angiogenesis.

Prolactin is most active during periods of pregnancy, where it leads to breast growth and mammary gland milk production. The regulation of PRL secretion is largely controlled via the inhibitory effects of dopamine, although thyrotropin-releasing hormone (TRH) also contributes and is able to directly stimulate release. Central serotonin also shows a stimulatory effect on PRL secretion. Prolactin exhibits mild gonadotropic effects and sensitizes luteinizing hormone (LH) receptors in Leydig cells, thereby increasing T production. Both T and PRL are subsequently able to suppress gonadotropin releasing hormone (GnRH), thereby helping to maintain appropriate PRL homeostatic levels.

The specific mechanism by which hyperprolactinemia causes low T has not been definitively described, although it likely includes both direct and indirect contributions. The presence of a pituitary adenoma (secreting or non-secreting) may result in suppression of GnRH/LH or destruction of GnRH/LH producing cells with subsequent declines in T production. Additionally, as a mild gonadotroph, PRL may feed back directly to the pituitary, resulting in the suppression of LH and T. Of note, from a purely diagnostic standpoint, true hyperprolactinemia occurs in the absence of macroprolactinemia, which may otherwise result in elevated prolactin levels without associated symptoms. The differentiation between these two conditions and diagnostic testing are beyond the scope of this chapter.

4.3   Clinical Symptoms and Prevalence
of Hyperprolactinemia in Men

Symptoms related to hyperprolactinemia may be due to the effect of PRL itself, suppression of other hormones (e.g., T), or a mass effect from a PRL-secreting mass. See Table 4.1 for a summary of common presenting symptoms in men with hyperprolactinemia. In a recent study evaluating the presenting symptoms of 28 elderly males (>65 year old) who were diagnosed with hyperprolactinemia, 61% complained of sexual dysfunction (e.g., low libido and erectile dysfunction [ED]), while 36% had no symptoms and were incidentally diagnosed [1]. Interestingly, only 7% complained of headaches or visual disturbances due to the mass effect from an underlying pituitary tumor. In contrast, in men who have large prolactinomas (defined as ≥40 mm diameter or ≥ 20 mm of suprasellar extension), visual

Table 4.1 Common presenting symptoms in men with hyperprolactinemia

Symptoms*	Frequencies
Sexual dysfunction (e.g., low libido and erectile dysfunction)	61%
Incidental finding (asymptomatic)	39%
Headache	7%
Visual disturbances	7%
Gynecomastia	Unknown (likely <5%)
Galactorrhea	Unknown (likely <5%)

*Symptoms as identified in men aged >65 [1]

disturbances are reported in up to 65% of cases [2]. This important finding highlights that earlier detection at the sexual dysfunction stage may prevent progression to a more advanced condition. Other symptoms such as gynecomastia or galactorrhea seldom occur with hyperprolactinemia in men, although the exact frequency with which they occur is unknown and is likely low.

In a series of men presenting to a sexual medicine clinic with varied sexual medicine complaints, a prevalence of mild elevations in prolactin (20–35 ng/mL) was found in 3.3%, while that of higher elevations (>35 ng/mL) was observed in 1.5% [3]. After controlling for low testosterone, TSH levels, and psychotropic drugs, higher prolactin levels remained significantly associated with low libido (HR 8.6). Similarly, following appropriate treatment of the elevated prolactin, libido improved at 6-month follow-up.

The prevalence of hyperprolactinemia in men with low T has not been well established. In contrast, majority of men with hyperprolactinemia are found to have low T. In a study of men >65 years old, 75% were found to have low T, while a second study of men aged 22–78 identified similarly high rates of low T (86%) [1, 4]. As noted earlier, this high rate of concomitant sexual dysfunction as well as sexual symptoms being the most common initial complaint of men with hyperprolactinemia suggests an essential role for the sexual medicine physician in appropriately identifying this condition through selective testing.

4.4   Etiologies for Hyperprolactinemia

Several different conditions and substances have been associated with hyperprolactinemia, including tumors, comorbid conditions, and medications, among others. See Table 4.2 for a more complete list of potential etiologies. Although pituitary tumors are relatively uncommon in men with low T, among those who are found to have hyperprolactinemia, they represent the most common single etiology and account for 41% of cases [5]. Other common causes included seizures (17%), medications (15%), acute illness (14%), chronic kidney disease (11%), transient (10%), and idiopathic (3%).

Table 4.2 Causes of hyperprolactinemia

Categories	Factors
Physiological	Sexual activity, exercise, sleep, stress
Hypothalamic-pituitary issues	Hypothalamic-pituitary stalk damage, acromegaly, lymphocytic hypophysitis, parasellar mass, prolactinoma, adenoma, surgery, trauma, radiation
Comorbid conditions	Chronic renal failure, cirrhosis, seizures
Medications	Antipsychotics (less with aripiprazole), bowel promotility agents (metoclopramide), tramadol, anesthetics, anticonvulsants, antidepressants (tricyclics, monoamine oxidase inhibitors, selective serotonin reuptake inhibitors, nefazodone, venlafaxine), antihistamines (H2), antihypertensives (verapamil)

In the majority of cases, management of the underlying cause for hyperprolactinemia typically leads to normalization of PRL levels. For example, among men with prolactin-secreting tumors, medical treatment with dopamine agonists resulted in normal PRL levels in 86% of individuals [1]. Similarly, men with chronic kidney disease and hyperprolactinemia who undergo renal transplantation experience subsequent declines in PRL levels [6].

In contrast to the above examples, medication-associated hyperprolactinemia is less well defined, and relatively limited data are available. The most common medication class implicated in hyperprolactinemia is anti-dopaminergic agents, including antipsychotics, with first-generation drugs being most commonly associated. More recent, second-generation agents have lesser impacts on PRL levels, which is thought to be secondary to combined dopamine agonist and antagonist properties (e.g., aripiprazole) [7]. However, this traditional concept of antipsychotic medication use being the sole cause of hyperprolactinemia has recently been called into questions. In a study of men with schizophrenia, 56% were found to have concomitant hyperprolactinemia at baseline, prior to antipsychotic use [8]. More recent data further supports this concept and suggests that the underlying psychotic disorder may actually contribute more to hyperprolactinemia than the antipsychotic medications themselves [9]. Furthermore, PRL levels may positively correlate with the severity of underlying psychosis. It is also unclear if drug substitution that results in lower PRL levels is due to the effects of the drug themselves, lesser effects of newer generation antipsychotics, or is indicative of improved underlying disease control [10]. Interestingly, in the above-mentioned study, among those who complained of concomitant sexual dysfunction, 92% were found to have elevated PRL levels compared to only 18% among those without sexual symptoms. The findings again highlight the interconnected nature and important predictive value of sexual symptoms in diagnosing hyperprolactinemia.

Other medications that have been associated with hyperprolactinemia include tramadol, verapamil, anti-dopaminergic bowel promotility agents (including metoclopramide), and select antidepressants (tricyclics, monoamine oxidase inhibitors, selective serotonin reuptake inhibitors, nefazodone, and venlafaxine) [11–13]

Primary hypothyroidism is also associated with hyperprolactinemia, likely due to reflexively elevated TRH levels. Although PRL typically improves with normalization of thyroid hormone, hyperprolactinemia has been reported even in the absence of overt thyroid hormone alterations (i.e., subclinical hypothyroidism) [14]. Hypothyroidism can be readily tested by obtaining a thyroid stimulating hormone (TSH) level. If this is elevated, it is suggestive of hypothyroidism and warrants referral to an endocrinologist for further management.

4.5   When to Obtain Prolactin Testing

The appropriate management of men with low T includes obtaining PRL levels in select clinical scenarios. The American Urological Association (AUA) and Endocrine Society guidelines on T deficiency both recommend obtaining PRL in men with low T and low/low-normal LH [15, 16]. From a physiologic standpoint, if LH is in the normal range, then this suggests the ability of the pituitary to release LH to stimulate the testicles and indicates that PRL testing is not required. In contrast, if LH is low or low/normal in the setting of low T, then this represents an inappropriate response and indicates a need to evaluate for potential causes of the hypogonadotropic hypogonadism. In a related manner, men with total T levels <150 ng/dl and low/low-normal LH should undergo a pituitary MRI regardless of PRL levels, given the possibility for non-PRL-secreting adenomas and higher yield at T levels <150 ng/dl [17].

In a 2016 publication summarizing recommendations from the Fourth International Consultation for Sexual Medicine (ICSM), Corona and colleagues suggested that clinicians should evaluate prolactin levels in all men complaining of decreased sexual desire (Recommendation #4) [18]. These recommendations were based on two studies which identified low libido in approximately 84% of individuals with prolactin levels >35 ng/dl, with two-thirds of these individuals exhibiting secondary pathology related to the elevated prolactin [3, 19]. However, <1 to 1% of individuals complaining of low libido were subsequently found to have notably elevated prolactin, suggesting that universal testing among all men with low libido may be of relatively low yield. Additionally, the number of men who had elevated prolactin in the absence of low testosterone or other associated symptoms was not reported, which likely represents an even smaller cohort. The authors did report that prolactin >35 ng/dl was associated with low libido, independent of hypogonadism; however, given the low overall yield, the role of universal prolactin testing in all men with low libido is debatable at the present time.

The interpretation of PRL and what is considered normal are not well established, and significant debate remains on optimal investigational and treatment thresholds. From a practicality standpoint, PRL levels <50 ng/ml are rarely associated with significant pathology, while higher levels (>250 ng/ml) are positively correlated with increasing likelihood for identifiable intracranial pathology, and levels >500 ng/ml are diagnostic of macroprolactinoma [2, 5, 20]. However, in the absence of better data, levels above normal thresholds, but lower than <50, should not prevent an investigation as to underlying causes or preclude treatment in the setting of hypogonadotropic hypogonadism.

Although transient elevations in PRL are not uncommon, the Endocrine Society does not recommend repeat or confirmatory testing in most cases of hyperprolactinemia [21].

4.6 Management of Hyperprolactinemia

As the target audience of this chapter is a non-endocrinologist practicing clinician, a complete and thorough description on the management of hyperprolactinemia is beyond the intended scope. In most cases, practicing clinicians will likely refer patients with elevated PRL to an endocrinology provider, which is consistent with AUA guideline recommendations [15]. However, a brief summary of general treatment strategies will be reviewed to provide a greater level of understanding, given that the initial diagnosis of hyperprolactinemia still relies on the sexual medicine provider. Each of the strategies noted below is based on the Endocrine Society Guideline on hyperprolactinemia [21]. See Fig. 4.1 for a proposed summary algorithm of the evaluation and treatment of hyperprolactinemia.

One of the first steps in managing hyperprolactinemia is to determine who does and does not merit treatment. Men with medication-induced hyperprolactinemia may be considered for medication substitution/trial of discontinuation if clinically viable. If this is not feasible, men with medication-induced hyperprolactinemia and low T (with associated symptoms/findings) are not recommended to undergo dopamine agonist therapies (e.g., cabergoline), but rather be treated with T directly. In cases of symptomatic hyperprolactinemia secondary to medications where the medication cannot be stopped, cautious consideration of a dopamine agonist may be elected.

Similarly, men with asymptomatic microprolactinomas are generally not recommended to be treated with dopamine agonists. In contrast, men with symptomatic microprolactinomas or macroprolactinomas (with or without symptoms) are appropriate for treatment.

Once the decision for therapy has been made, dopaminergic agents such as cabergoline are recommended as first-line agents. Initiation of cabergoline leads to normalization of PRL levels in 71–86% and tumor shrinkage in approximately 80% of men [1, 22]. Those with smaller microadenomas may experience even higher success rates (95%) [23]. In men who are resistant to cabergoline (approximately 10%), bromocriptine may be substituted.

Once successful treatment has been achieved for at least 2 years (normalized PRL levels and no visible tumor), therapy may be tapered off with subsequent biochemical follow-up. In men who do not respond, maximally tolerated dosing of dopamine agonists is recommended prior to consideration of surgery.

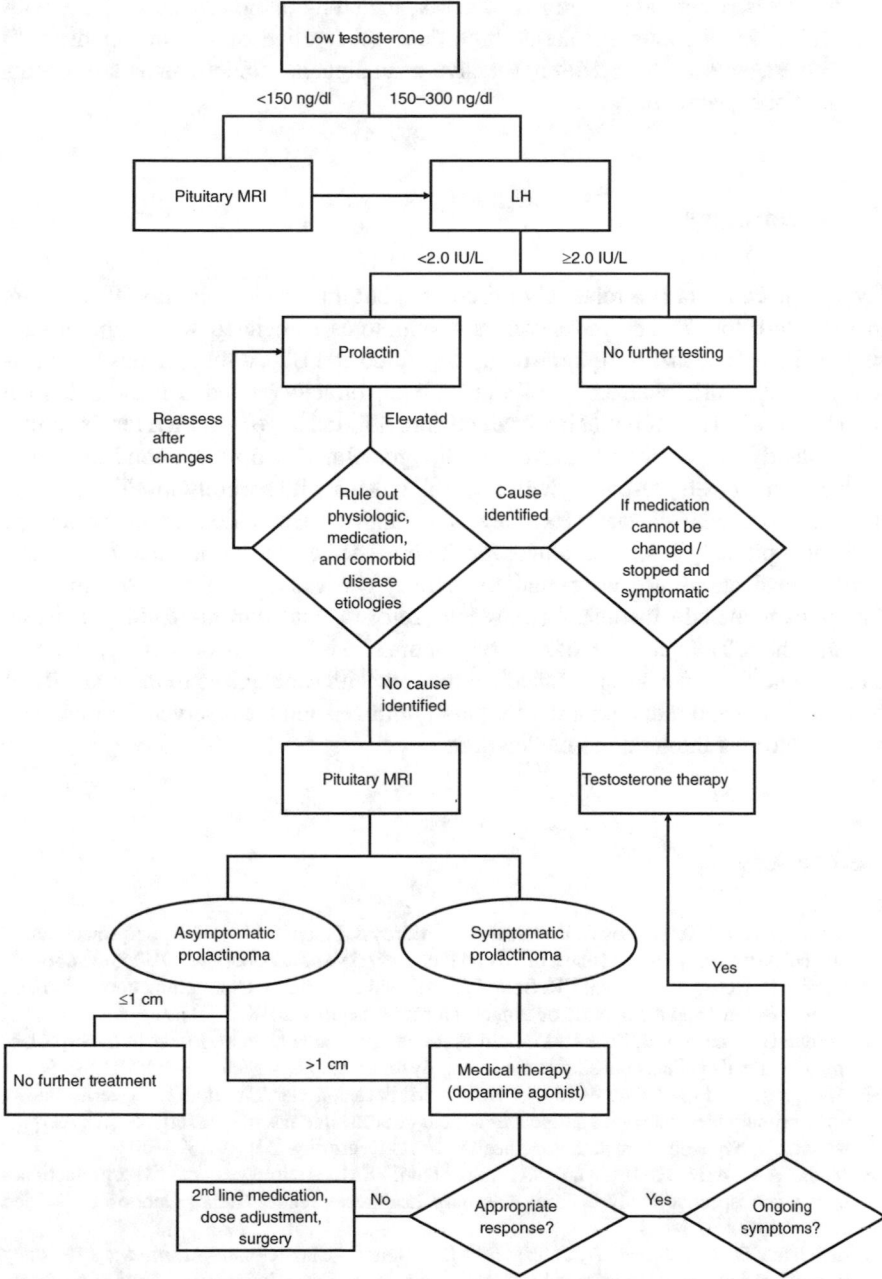

Fig. 4.1 Proposed algorithm for the evaluation and management of low testosterone as it relates to prolactin and hyperprolactinemia

Surgery is recommended in select cases, including symptomatic patients with prolactinomas who cannot tolerate high-dose cabergoline or are unresponsive to dopamine agonists. Those with aggressive or malignant prolactinomas are recommended for radiation therapy.

4.7 Summary

Hyperprolactinemia is a relatively infrequent, but important, condition that occurs in men with low T. The most common symptoms associated with hyperprolactinemia include sexual symptoms (e.g., low libido and ED), although these are relatively indistinguishable from low T and are likely directly related to T levels. In men with low T, a LH level should be obtained and, if found to be low, PRL levels should subsequently be performed. Current ICSM guidelines also recommend obtaining prolactin in all men presenting with low libido. Men with severely low T (<150 ng/dl) and those with elevated PRL levels without a clearly defined cause should undergo a pituitary MRI to evaluate for the presence of micro- or macroadenomas. Further evaluations are warranted to identify the cause of hyperprolactinemia, which may include medications, hypothyroidism, and chronic kidney disease, among others. The treatment of hyperprolactinemia is typically best managed by an endocrinologist and consists of medical therapy with cabergoline in the majority of cases. Surgery and radiation are infrequently utilized and are reserved for men who are refractory or intolerant to medications.

References

1. Shimon I, Hirsch D, Tsvetov G, Robenshtok E, Akirov A, Fraenkel M, et al. Hyperprolactinemia diagnosis in elderly men: a cohort of 28 patients over 65 years. Endocrine. 2019;65(3):656–61.
2. Iglesias P, Arcano K, Berrocal VR, Bernal C, Villabona C, Diez JJ. Giant prolactinoma in men: clinical features and therapeutic outcomes. Horm Metab Res. 2018;50(11):791–6.
3. Corona G, Mannucci E, Fisher AD, Lotti F, Ricca V, Balercia G, et al. Effect of hyperprolactinemia in male patients consulting for sexual dysfunction. J Sex Med. 2007;4(5):1485–93.
4. Andereggen L, Frey J, Andres RH, El-Koussy M, Beck J, Seiler RW, et al. Long-term follow-up of primary medical versus surgical treatment of prolactinomas in men: effects on hyperprolactinemia, hypogonadism, and bone health. World Neurosurg. 2017;97:595–602.
5. Malik AA, Aziz F, Beshyah SA, Aldahmani KM. Aetiologies of hyperprolactinaemia: a retrospective analysis from a tertiary healthcare centre. Sultan Qaboos Univ Med J. 2019;19(2):e129–e34.
6. Eckersten D, Giwercman A, Pihlsgard M, Bruun L, Christensson A. Impact of kidney transplantation on reproductive hormone levels in males: a longitudinal study. Nephron. 2018;138(3):192–201.
7. Saitis M, Papazisis G, Katsigiannopoulos K, Kouvelas D. Aripiprazole resolves amisulpride and ziprasidone-induced hyperprolactinemia. Psychiatry Clin Neurosci. 2008;62(5):624.

8. Zhang Y, Tang Z, Ruan Y, Huang C, Wu J, Lu Z, et al. Prolactin and thyroid stimulating hormone (TSH) levels and sexual dysfunction in patients with schizophrenia treated with conventional antipsychotic medication: a cross-sectional study. Med Sci Monit. 2018;24:9136–43.
9. Vuk Pisk S, Matic K, Geres N, Ivezic E, Ruljancic N, Filipcic I. Hyperprolactinemia – side effect or part of the illness. Psychiatr Danub. 2019;31(Suppl 2):148–52.
10. Nunes LV, Moreira HC, Razzouk D, Nunes SO, Mari JJ. Strategies for the treatment of antipsychotic-induced sexual dysfunction and/or hyperprolactinemia among patients of the schizophrenia spectrum: a review. J Sex Marital Ther. 2012;38(3):281–301.
11. Gluskin LE, Strasberg B, Shah JH. Verapamil-induced hyperprolactinemia and galactorrhea. Ann Intern Med. 1981;95(1):66–7.
12. Molitch ME. Medication-induced hyperprolactinemia. Mayo Clin Proc. 2005;80(8):1050–7.
13. Farag AGA, Basha MA, Amin SA, Elnaidany NF, Elhelbawy NG, Mostafa MMT, et al. Tramadol (opioid) abuse is associated with a dose- and time-dependent poor sperm quality and hyperprolactinaemia in young men. Andrologia. 2018;50(6):e13026.
14. Aziz K, Shahbaz A, Umair M, Sharifzadeh M, Sachmechi I. Hyperprolactinemia with galactorrhea due to subclinical hypothyroidism: a case report and review of literature. Cureus. 2018;10(5):e2723.
15. Mulhall JP, Trost LW, Brannigan RE, Kurtz EG, Redmon JB, Chiles KA, et al. Evaluation and management of testosterone deficiency: AUA guideline. J Urol. 2018;200(2):423–32.
16. Bhasin S, Brito JP, Cunningham GR, Hayes FJ, Hodis HN, Matsumoto AM, et al. Testosterone therapy in men with hypogonadism: an Endocrine Society clinical practice guideline. J Clin Endocrinol Metab. 2018;103(5):1715–44.
17. Citron JT, Ettinger B, Rubinoff H, Ettinger VM, Minkoff J, Hom F, et al. Prevalence of hypothalamic-pituitary imaging abnormalities in impotent men with secondary hypogonadism. J Urol. 1996;155(2):529–33.
18. Corona G, Isidori AM, Aversa A, Burnett AL, Maggi M. Endocrinologic control of men's sexual desire and arousal/erection. J Sex Med. 2016;13(3):317–37.
19. Corona G, Rastrelli G, Ricca V, Jannini EA, Vignozzi L, Monami M, et al. Risk factors associated with primary and secondary reduced libido in male patients with sexual dysfunction. J Sex Med. 2013;10(4):1074–89.
20. Vilar L, Freitas MC, Naves LA, Casulari LA, Azevedo M, Montenegro R Jr, et al. Diagnosis and management of hyperprolactinemia: results of a Brazilian multicenter study with 1234 patients. J Endocrinol Investig. 2008;31(5):436–44.
21. Melmed S, Casanueva FF, Hoffman AR, Kleinberg DL, Montori VM, Schlechte JA, et al. Diagnosis and treatment of hyperprolactinemia: an Endocrine Society clinical practice guideline. J Clin Endocrinol Metab. 2011;96(2):273–88.
22. Berinder K, Stackenas I, Akre O, Hirschberg AL, Hulting AL. Hyperprolactinaemia in 271 women: up to three decades of clinical follow-up. Clin Endocrinol. 2005;63(4):450–5.
23. Webster J, Piscitelli G, Polli A, D'Alberton A, Falsetti L, Ferrari C, et al. Dose-dependent suppression of serum prolactin by cabergoline in hyperprolactinaemia: a placebo controlled, double blind, multicentre study. European Multicentre Cabergoline Dose-finding Study Group. Clin Endocrinol. 1992;37(6):534–41.

Chapter 5
Testosterone and Disordered Sleep

Fiona Yuen, Bahman Chavoshan, Danya Waqfi, and Peter Y. Liu

5.1 Introduction

In the past few decades, our knowledge of the role that sleep exerts on many aspects of health has expanded significantly. Disordered sleep has been shown to negatively impact cardiometabolic health, diminish psychomotor performance, and affect multiple other physiological functions that are pertinent to men's health. Disordered sleep may be restricted or insufficient (decreased total sleep time), misaligned to the endogenous circadian rhythm (as may be seen in night shift workers), or disrupted (as occurs with nocturia or obstructive sleep apnea). Insufficient, misaligned, and disrupted sleep has distinct effects on sleep architecture. Since each sleep stage

---

F. Yuen · D. Waqfi
Division of Endocrinology, Department of Medicine, The Lundquist Institute at Harbor-UCLA Medical Center, Torrance, CA, USA

B. Chavoshan
Department of Graduate Medical Education, St. Mary Medical Center,
Long Beach, CA, USA

David Geffen School of Medicine, University of California, Los Angeles,
Los Angeles, CA, USA

P. Y. Liu (✉)
Division of Endocrinology, Department of Medicine, The Lundquist Institute at Harbor-UCLA Medical Center, Torrance, CA, USA

David Geffen School of Medicine, University of California, Los Angeles,
Los Angeles, CA, USA

David Geffen School of Medicine at UCLA, Division of Endocrinology and Metabolism, Department of Medicine, Harbor UCLA Medical Center and Los Angeles Biomedical Research Institute, Torrance, CA, USA
e-mail: pliu@lundquist.org

© Springer Nature Switzerland AG 2021
J. P. Mulhall et al. (eds.), *Controversies in Testosterone Deficiency*,
https://doi.org/10.1007/978-3-030-77111-9_5

serves specific physiological functions, insufficient, misaligned, and disrupted sleep could differentially influence different aspects of andrological and metabolic health. Conceptualizing this requires an understanding of normal sleep architecture.

The adult human sleep cycle is 90–120 minutes in duration. Sleep cycles are divided into non-rapid eye movement (NREM) and rapid eye movement (REM) sleep. Each stage of sleep can be recognized by characteristic electrophysiological features: specific waveforms and frequencies of brain activity on electroencephalogram (EEG), rolling or saccadic eye movements detected by electrooculogram, and skeletal muscle activity revealed by electromyography. NREM sleep contributes to 75–80% of total sleep time and is itself subdivided into three stages: N1, N2, and N3. N1 generally progresses to N3 as sleep deepens and waveform frequencies slow on the EEG. Stage 3 NREM sleep, also known as slow wave sleep (SWS), typically occurs during the first one-third of the night and is believed to be the most restorative type of sleep that underpins important metabolic processes, including restoring insulin sensitivity [1, 2]. During SWS, cerebral blood flow and metabolism are reduced. There is also increased secretion of growth hormone during SWS [1]. In contrast, REM sleep contributes to 20–25% of the total time spent in sleep, and REM cycles progressively lengthen as the night progresses [3]. REM sleep is required for memory consolidation and for sleep-related increase in systemic testosterone exposure [4].

Restricting sleep decreases total sleep time, but SWS tends to be maintained, so metabolic processes dependent on SWS such as insulin sensitivity may also be relatively preserved. Circadian misalignment of sleep may advance (initiating sleep earlier) or delay sleep (initiating sleep later). When sleep is advanced, SWS and REM are reduced. When sleep is delayed, N2 decreases, SWS is preserved, and REM sleep increases [5]. Disrupted sleep interrupts normal sleep architecture by interfering with the orderly progression of the sleep stages. Causes of disrupted sleep include environmental (e.g., light, noise, and bed partner movements) and pathologic (e.g., nocturia and OSA) factors. OSA may sometimes disrupt REM sleep in particular, when the collapsibility risk from reduced upper airway muscular tone is predominant. Accordingly, a reduction in systemic testosterone exposure with REM-associated OSA would be expected.

This chapter focuses on the effects of common causes of disordered sleep on andrological health, emphasizing well-established surrogates such as semen parameters for male fertility and circulating testosterone concentrations for hypogonadism.

5.2   Insufficient Sleep

It is recommended that adults aged 18–64 years sleep 8 hours per night on average, although the restorative amount of sleep ranges from 7 to 9 hours each night for any particular individual [6]. Despite these recommendations, over a third of American adults report insufficient sleep durations on a regular basis [7]. Some causes of insufficient sleep include lifestyle and environmental factors, such as shift work, noise, prolonged working hours, and jet lag; other causes include sleep disorders such as insomnia and other medical conditions [3]. Insufficient sleep is linked to increased mortality, andrological and cardiovascular disease, and metabolic disorders including diabetes mellitus. Interventional studies investigating the effects of restricting sleep reveal worsened insulin resistance and increased blood pressure, especially nocturnal blood pressure [8].

5.2.1   Effect on Reproductive Health

Carefully conducted in-laboratory studies have shown that testosterone levels rise during sleep and disruption of the normal sleep architecture prevents this rise in testosterone [9]. Epidemiological studies have explored the relationship between sleep duration and testosterone. However, findings from epidemiological cohort studies have not been consistent. Some studies reveal lower testosterone levels with shorter durations of self-reported sleep, while other studies do not [8]. It may be that only sleep loss occurring during the second half of the night actually reduces testosterone levels [10]. This hypothesis, if correct, could explain the inconsistent findings from observational studies because the timing of sleep loss has not been considered. On the other hand, carefully controlled in-laboratory interventional studies have consistently shown that sleep restriction decreases testosterone [10–12], including a recent study showing for the first time that sleep restriction decreases testosterone levels in older men [13]. This novel finding raises the possibility that sleep loss accumulated over decades of life in older men may contribute to age-related hypoandrogenemia [14].

Epidemiological studies have also explored the relationship between sleep duration and male fertility. One study showed that in 1176 couples planning a pregnancy, male partners who self-reported sleeping <6 hour each night had lower conception rates [15]. However, it is difficult to know whether it was the male or the female partner's sleep that was actually responsible for reduced conception rates as bed partners may have similar sleeping patterns. Two studies of healthy young men found associations between sleep and semen parameters. One study of healthy, young Danish men showed that either low or high self-reported sleep quality was associated with lower sperm concentrations, lower total sperm count, and a decrease in the percent of sperm motility and morphologically normal spermatozoa, compared with those who reported mid-levels of sleep quality [16]. This study did not investigate sleep duration, and it is difficult to understand why both low- and high-quality sleep would be associated with poorer semen parameters. A second study in Chinese men, primarily military cadets, found that men who self-reported sleep durations of <6.5 hours or >9.0 hours had lower total sperm count and semen volume [17]. Sperm chromatin was less mature, but there was no significant effect on DNA fragmentation [18]. In a subset of these men who supplied semen samples 1 year later, a significant increase in total sperm count was observed in those who shifted their sleep away from extreme durations toward a hypothesized ideal duration of 7–7.5 hours/night [17]. However, this study relied on self-reported sleep durations, the analysis appeared ad hoc, and the reasons for the improvement in sleep were not determined. In animal studies, male rats that underwent sleep deprivation for 96 continuous hours or partial sleep restriction (<6 hours/night) for 21 nights had lower sperm viability and elevated endothelial nitric oxide synthase expression compared to controls [19]. Another study also showed a decrease in sperm motility in rats that underwent 7 days of continuous sleep deprivation compared to controls [20]. A third study found a decrease in sperm count, motility and morphology, as well as decreased viability, in those rats that underwent 5 days of continuous sleep deprivation compared to controls [21]. The investigators also noted increased testicular gene expression of nuclear factor kappa beta (NF-κβ) and decreased nuclear factor-like 2 (Nrf2) expression. NF-κβ is involved in activating nitric oxide synthase, and Nrf2 is involved in regulating glutathione. Together, these findings suggest that sleep restriction affects semen quality, plausibly by increasing oxidative stress.

Two studies have also shown cross-sectional, inverse U-shaped relationships between sleep (quality or duration) and lower testicular volume in humans. In the aforementioned study of young Danish men, those who reported high (and low) levels of sleep quality had lower testicular size [16]. The other study using home actigraphy to objectively determine sleep onset and wake time, along with self-reported sleep duration and quality, showed an inverse U-shaped correlation only between sleep duration and testicular volume [22].

Longitudinal observational studies that examine the effects of sleep disturbances on changes in conception rates and testicular volumes have yet to be performed. To establish a direct relationship between sleep restriction and fertility rates, an interventional study might require sleep restriction for over 3 months, given that the spermatogenic cycle is 3 months in duration. Such an interventional study would be a major undertaking.

5.3   Misaligned Sleep

Every cell, tissue, and organ in the body contains a molecular clock. These peripheral clocks are synchronized by the master circadian pacemaker which lies in the suprachiasmatic nucleus (SCN) of the hypothalamus through hormonal (melatonin, and cortisol for metabolically active organs) and autonomic signals. The master circadian pacemaker is composed of specific neurons in the SCN that are coupled together through direct cell-to-cell connections. These neurons generate autonomous circadian rhythms which oscillate with a periodicity that is slightly greater than 24 hours. Accordingly, the master circadian pacemaker needs to be entrained to the environmental day/night cycle on a daily basis through external cues known as *zeitgebers* ("time-givers," from German) to remain aligned with the environmental day. Unsurprisingly, the main *zeitgeber* is light, and SCN neurons receive direct photic inputs from the retina for this purpose, which are distinct from the visual processing system [23, 24]. Other *zeitgebers* include personal and societal patterns of eating and physical activity.

Common causes of misaligned sleep include jetlag (fast trans-meridian travel) and certain work schedules (night and alternating shift work). Shift work in particular has been linked to multiple adverse health outcomes. Workers who sleep during the day are sleeping during the normal wake phase of their biological rhythms. They often also experience environmental factors such as light and noise at inappropriate times that further adversely impact the duration and quality of sleep and may also voluntarily wake up earlier to interact with family members, thus further curtailing the total sleep time. Shift work has been linked to lower performance and increased industrial incidents (e.g., Chernobyl nuclear disaster); cardiometabolic diseases such as diabetes mellitus, obesity, hypertension, and ischemic heart disease; as well as overall mortality [25]. These epidemiological studies cannot establish a definitive causal relationship between shift work and adverse health outcomes, however. On the other hand, interventional studies that misalign sleep under highly controlled laboratory conditions have demonstrated worsening of well-established markers of cardiometabolic health, such as insulin resistance and systemic blood pressure, thereby suggesting a causal link [8].

5.3.1 Effect on Reproductive Health

Epidemiological studies show that shift work in the male partner does not impair fertility if there is no actual sleep loss [26–28]. Several of these studies did find that male infertility was associated with higher levels of physical exertion and psychological stress but not with shift work [27]. Many of these studies were conducted in fertility clinics, and thus their participants may not be representative of the general population. Other epidemiological studies also did not find a significant difference in semen parameters with shift work [29, 30]. There are no randomized studies that investigate the relationship between misaligned sleep and semen parameters.

Epidemiological studies have also investigated the relationship between shift work and testosterone levels. However, these studies of clinic populations or of workplace employees may not be representative of the population as a whole. A study of men seen in an andrology clinic found that among men working nonstandard shifts, those who reported better sleep quality had fewer hypogonadal symptoms and superior sexual function. Blood testosterone levels were also measured in these men. However, over 40% of the men were receiving testosterone therapy or medications that alter systemic testosterone levels (such as clomiphene, anastrozole, or human chorionic gonadotropin) [31].

Other studies in the workplace investigated testosterone levels in the saliva or blood but did not measure samples over the entire day. One workplace study found no change in salivary testosterone levels in rotating shift workers examined during a night shift schedule or during a recovery day shift schedule [32]. This study did not obtain salivary testosterone levels during sleep. A small study in junior physicians undergoing a rotating shift work schedule also found no change in testosterone levels when examined after a holiday, or after day shift and night shift conditions. Only one time point was assessed for each of the three conditions and the time of blood draw was not specified [33]. As testosterone levels vary widely during the day, a single time point will not provide a complete picture, especially if the time of awakening is unknown. Another small study found that the overall mean concentration of testosterone in shift workers was less than that of controls. However, blood draws occurred only during the night when the night shift workers were awake and the day shift worker controls were asleep [34]. Since testosterone rises during sleep, mean testosterone levels would be expected to be lower in the awake night shift workers compared with the asleep day shift workers, when only nighttime, not 24-hour, testosterone levels are assessed.

In fact, only one study has examined 24-hour testosterone exposure in the workplace. This study reported numerically higher 24-hour levels of urinary androgens and higher 24-hour levels of urinary testosterone in male night shift workers compared to male day shift workers. However, 24-hour urinary androgens and urinary testosterone were not statistically different between these day and night shift workers [35].

Whereas the prior studies were performed in a workplace setting, there is however one study that was conducted in a highly controlled laboratory environment. In this study, normal young men who were not selected on the basis of being habitual shift workers underwent a shift work schedule of nighttime wake or daytime wake in a balanced cross-over design in order to examine blood testosterone levels. No difference in 24-hour mean testosterone levels was observed, implying that the acute (1 day) shift in work schedule did not alter overall systemic testosterone concentrations. It did, however, find that testosterone levels rose with sleep and fell during wakefulness, irrespective of whether sleep occurred during the day or night [36].

In summary, there does not appear to be a significant change in mean testosterone levels with circadian misalignment due to shift work. However, this conclusion is based almost entirely on observational studies in actual shift workers. Most did not examine 24-hour testosterone exposure and were likely affected by sampling bias and other confounders. Furthermore, the single in-laboratory interventional study did not impose a realistic shift work schedule, nor was it designed to be able to fully separate changes in testosterone due to sleep from those due to circadian misalignment. Nevertheless, the diurnal rhythm of testosterone appears to be dependent upon sleep (regardless of whether it occurs during the day or night), and testosterone levels are therefore highest shortly after awakening. The Endocrine Society recommends measuring testosterone in the early morning on two separate occasions to assess for hypogonadism [37] and does not specify when testosterone should be measured in shift workers. Based on this review, testosterone should be measured soon after awakening, not necessarily in the early morning, in shift workers. This is to obtain blood levels that are most comparable with the standard testosterone reference range applied to non-shift workers.

5.4 Disrupted Sleep

Many medical conditions disrupt sleep. Perhaps the most common cause is obstructive sleep apnea (OSA). Nocturia, due to prostatic problems or diuretic use, is also a common cause. Other causes include poorly controlled asthma, heart failure, and gastroesophageal reflux disease. In OSA, recurring partial closure of the pharyngeal airway occurs during sleep leading to decreased airflow (hypopnea) or complete cessation of breath (apnea). This leads to hypercapnia and hypoxemia, causing the patient to arouse. OSA presents more commonly in men than in women and the prevalence of OSA increases with age. With the current obesity epidemic, it is estimated that 13% of men and 6% of women have moderate to severe sleep-disordered breathing [38]. OSA is treatable with the application of continuous positive airway pressure (CPAP) therapy. Epidemiological studies have shown that OSA increases the risk of all-cause mortality, type 2 diabetes mellitus, systemic hypertension, and coronary artery disease. Interventional trials have shown that effective CPAP improves cardiovascular parameters including blood pressure and ventricular ejection fraction and also decreases cardiac dysrhythmias. However, a clear decrease in cardiovascular mortality has not been evident [39]. Given the negative impact of sleep disruption on overall health, the underlying medical causes should be optimally treated.

5.4.1 Effects on Reproductive Health

There are no data from large-scale epidemiological studies linking OSA with male fertility. Interventional trials have demonstrated the relationship between OSA and erectile dysfunction, and most trials have shown improvement in erectile function and sexual satisfaction with treatment of OSA [8]. The only randomized sham-controlled trial reported that CPAP can improve erectile function but only if men are compliant with CPAP use [40]. No studies have been performed to examine the effects of OSA or reversal of CPAP on semen parameters or fertility in men. However, an animal study found that mice subjected to periodic hypoxia for 60 days had a decreased proportion of pregnant females per mating, decreased sperm motility, and increased markers of testicular oxidative stress [41].

Epidemiological studies link more severe OSA to lower testosterone levels, but it is not certain whether this relationship is or is not related to concomitant obesity [8]. Furthermore, many of the symptoms of OSA overlap with those of hypogonadism. The effects of OSA treatment on testosterone levels are also controversial. Although a recent meta-analysis concluded that CPAP does not increase systemic testosterone levels [42], this conclusion may not be warranted if only higher quality studies are examined. The authors recognized that only two of the studies included in the meta-analysis were randomized: one of these studies randomized between two different treatments of OSA and so was unable to capitalize on randomization to assess the effect of treatment of OSA alone [43]. Furthermore, combining studies that have methodological or design flaws by meta-analysis does not overcome the original limitations. In contrast, when examining higher quality studies, the three most notable studies have each concluded that treatment of OSA increases testosterone. The first study is the only study utilizing a randomized sham-controlled design. It reported that those randomized to CPAP had greater increases in testosterone compared with those randomized to sham – but the difference between groups was due to a fall in testosterone in the sham group [44]. The second study is the only study that assessed testosterone exposure frequently over an extended period of time (every 20 minutes from 7 PM to 7 AM). A significant increase in testosterone after 9 months of CPAP was reported; however, only five highly CPAP-adherent men were studied [45]. Nevertheless, all other studies have assessed one or two time points, usually in the morning. The third study was the only study where near-complete reversal of sleep-disordered breathing was achieved [46]. This study reported an increase in morning testosterone levels after 3 months of therapy in 12 men, but the intervention was surgical uvulopalatopharyngoplasty, not CPAP. Accordingly, it may be that adherent CPAP therapy is needed to increase testosterone. However, large-scale studies are yet to be performed, and the overall data currently do not allow firm conclusions to be drawn.

5.4.2   Testosterone Replacement Therapy and Obstructive Sleep Apnea

Testosterone therapy is widely believed to induce or worsen sleep apnea, but the evidence that underpins this relationship is weak [37]. Nevertheless, two randomized controlled trials do show that testosterone therapy can acutely induce sleep-disordered breathing. One of the studies resulted in levels of testosterone that were definitely supraphysiological due to the dose administered [47] and the other likely induced supraphysiological peaks due to the drug pharmacokinetics of short ester-chain testosterone intramuscular injections [48]. Whether these adverse findings would occur with longer-term near-physiological testosterone replacement, as now occurs in clinical practice with modern testosterone formulations, is uncertain.

Two other randomized, placebo-controlled, parallel group studies have partly filled this gap in knowledge by investigating the effect of longer-term replacement dose and more steady-state testosterone therapy on sleep-disordered breathing [49, 50]. The first study administered a dose-titrated testosterone patch ($n = 54$) or a matching dose-titrated placebo patch ($n = 54$) to healthy men over the age of 65 for 3 years [49]. The initial dose was 6 mg/day, which was adjusted every 3 months to maintain blood testosterone levels below 1000 ng/dL. No significant difference between the two groups was detected after 6, 12, 24, or 36 months of therapy; however, sleep-disordered breathing was assessed at home with a relatively insensitive portable instrument which may not have detected the development of mild or moderate OSA. The second study is the only study to purposefully administer testosterone to men with known moderate to severe OSA. Obese men with OSA received three doses of testosterone undecanoate 1000 mg every 6 weeks ($n = 33$), or matching placebo ($n = 34$), as well as a hypocaloric diet which caused weight loss that was comparable between the two groups [50]. The study reported that testosterone treatment significantly increased sleep-disordered breathing by a moderate amount (10 events/hour) at week 7 (1 week after the second injection of testosterone undecanoate), but not at week 18. Available studies suggest that sleep-disordered breathing occurs because testosterone affects ventilatory drive [51, 52]. A meta-analysis of 19 randomized controlled trials evaluating the effects of testosterone replacement therapy in hypogonadal men aged 45 and over on a range of outcomes did not find a significant difference in the incidence of OSA; however, only symptomatic severe OSA would have been reported since OSA was not systematically assessed by polysomnography so that effects on the apnea-hypopnea index (AHI) were not reported [53]. Overall, studies show some evidence that the initiation of testosterone therapy might induce or worsen OSA, but any effects are moderate in size and may not persist. Nevertheless, the Endocrine Society has made, for now, a prudent recommendation to avoid initiating testosterone therapy in those with untreated severe OSA [37].

5.5   Conclusion

Disordered sleep can be categorized as insufficient, misaligned, or disrupted. Epidemiological data have established a relationship between disordered sleep and increased mortality, cancer, cardiovascular disease, insulin resistance, and type 2 diabetes mellitus. This review shows that disordered sleep also affects andrological health: insufficient sleep decreases testosterone, whereas circadian misalignment due to shift work or simulated shift work schedule per se does not. Disrupted sleep due to obstructive sleep apnea is associated with lower systemic testosterone concentrations, although this may be due to concomitant adiposity. Preliminary data suggest the possibility that male fertility and semen parameters may also be impacted by sleep duration, but the impacts of circadian misalignment and/or disrupted sleep on fertility have not yet been studied comprehensively. In any case, sleep should be prioritized and valued to promote overall health, including andrological well-being. Methods to minimize deleterious effects of shift work and to promote CPAP adherence remain important research priorities.

References

1. Dijk DJ. Regulation and functional correlates of slow wave sleep. J Clin Sleep Med. 2009;5(2 Suppl):S6–15.
2. Tasali E, Leproult R, Ehrmann DA, Van Cauter E. Slow-wave sleep and the risk of type 2 diabetes in humans. Proc Natl Acad Sci U S A. 2008;105(3):1044–9.
3. Institute of Medicine (IOM). In: Colten HR, Altevogt BM, editors. Sleep disorders and sleep deprivation: an unmet public health problem. The National Academies Collection: reports funded by National Institutes of Health. Washington, DC: National Academies of Science; 2006.

4. Luboshitzky R, Zabari Z, Shen-Orr Z, Herer P, Lavie P. Disruption of the nocturnal testosterone rhythm by sleep fragmentation in normal men. J Clin Endocrinol Metab. 2001;86(3):1134–9.
5. Gonnissen HK, Hursel R, Rutters F, Martens EA, Westerterp-Plantenga MS. Effects of sleep fragmentation on appetite and related hormone concentrations over 24 h in healthy men. Br J Nutr. 2013;109(4):748–56. https://doi.org/10.1017/S0007114512001894.
6. Hirshkowitz M, Whiton K, Albert SM, Alessi C, Bruni O, DonCarlos L, et al. National Sleep Foundation's sleep time duration recommendations: methodology and results summary. Sleep Health. 2015;1(1):40–3. https://doi.org/10.1016/j.sleh.2014.12.010.
7. Liu Y, Wheaton AG, Chapman DP, Cunningham TJ, Lu H, Croft JB. Prevalence of healthy sleep duration among adults — United States, 2014. Morb Mortal Wkly Rep. 2016;65:137–41. https://doi.org/10.15585/mmwr.mm6506a1.
8. Liu PY. A clinical perspective of sleep and andrological health: assessment, treatment considerations and future research. J Clin Endocrinol Metab. 2019;104(10):4398–417. https://doi.org/10.1210/jc.2019-00683.
9. Luboshitzky R, Lavi S, Thuma I, Lavie P. Testosterone treatment alters melatonin concentrations in male patients with gonadotropin-releasing hormone deficiency. J Clin Endocrinol Metab. 1996;81(2):770–4.
10. Schmid SM, Hallschmid M, Jauch-Chara K, Lehnert H, Schultes B. Sleep timing may modulate the effect of sleep loss on testosterone. Clin Endocrinol. 2012;77(5):749–54. https://doi.org/10.1111/j.1365-2265.2012.04419.x.
11. Leproult R, Van Cauter E. Effect of 1 week of sleep restriction on testosterone levels in young healthy men. J Am Med Assoc. 2011;305(21):2173–4. https://doi.org/10.1001/jama.2011.710.
12. Reynolds AC, Dorrian J, Liu PY, Van Dongen HPA, Wittert GA, Harmer LJ, et al. Impact of five nights of sleep restriction on glucose metabolism, leptin and testosterone in young adult men. PLoS One. 2012;7(7):e41218. https://doi.org/10.1371/journal.pone.0041218.
13. Liu PY, Takahashi PY, Yang RJ, Iranmanesh A, Veldhuis JD. Age and time-of-day differences in the hypothalamo-pituitary-testicular, and adrenal, response to total overnight sleep deprivation. Sleep. 2020;43(7):zsaa008. https://doi.org/10.1093/sleep/zsaa008.
14. Liu PY, Takahashi P, Nehra A, Pincus SM, Keenan DM, Veldhuis JD. Neuroendocrine aging: pituitary–gonadal axis in males. In: Editor-in-Chief: Larry RS, editor. Encyclopedia of neuroscience. Oxford: Academic Press; 2009. p. 317–26.
15. Wise LA, Rothman KJ, Wesselink AK, Mikkelsen EM, Sorensen HT, McKinnon CJ, et al. Male sleep duration and fecundability in a North American preconception cohort study. Fertil Steril. 2018;109(3):453–9. https://doi.org/10.1016/j.fertnstert.2017.11.037.
16. Jensen TK, Andersson AM, Skakkebaek NE, Joensen UN, Blomberg Jensen M, Lassen TH, et al. Association of sleep disturbances with reduced semen quality: a cross-sectional study among 953 healthy young Danish men. Am J Epidemiol. 2013;177(10):1027–37. https://doi.org/10.1093/aje/kws420.
17. Chen Q, Yang H, Zhou N, Sun L, Bao H, Tan L, et al. Inverse U-shaped Association between sleep duration and semen quality: longitudinal observational study (MARHCS) in Chongqing, China. Sleep. 2016;39(1):79–86. https://doi.org/10.5665/sleep.5322.
18. Wang X, Chen Q, Zou P, Liu T, Mo M, Yang H, et al. Sleep duration is associated with sperm chromatin integrity among young men in Chongqing, China. J Sleep Res. 2018;27(4):e12615. https://doi.org/10.1111/jsr.12615.
19. Alvarenga TA, Hirotsu C, Mazaro-Costa R, Tufik S, Andersen ML. Impairment of male reproductive function after sleep deprivation. Fertil Steril. 2015;103(5):1355–62 e1. https://doi.org/10.1016/j.fertnstert.2015.02.002.
20. Choi JH, Lee SH, Bae JH, Shim JS, Park HS, Kim YS, et al. Effect of sleep deprivation on the male reproductive system in rats. J Korean Med Sci. 2016;31(10):1624–30. https://doi.org/10.3346/jkms.2016.31.10.1624.
21. Rizk NI, Rizk MS, Mohamed AS, Naguib YM. Attenuation of sleep deprivation dependent deterioration in male fertility parameters by vitamin C. Reprod Biol Endocrinol. 2020;18(1):2. https://doi.org/10.1186/s12958-020-0563-y.

22. Zhang W, Piotrowska K, Chavoshan B, Wallace J, Liu PY. Sleep duration is associated with testis size in healthy young men. J Clin Sleep Med. 2018;14(10):1757–64.
23. Reppert SM, Weaver DR. Coordination of circadian timing in mammals. Nature. 2002;418(6901):935–41. https://doi.org/10.1038/nature00965.
24. Welsh DK, Takahashi JS, Kay SA. Suprachiasmatic nucleus: cell autonomy and network properties. Annu Rev Physiol. 2010;72:551–77. https://doi.org/10.1146/annurev-physiol-021909-135919.
25. James SM, Honn KA, Gaddameedhi S, Van Dongen HPA. Shift work: disrupted circadian rhythms and sleep-implications for health and well-being. Curr Sleep Med Rep. 2017;3(2):104–12. https://doi.org/10.1007/s40675-017-0071-6.
26. Bisanti L, Olsen J, Basso O, Thonneau P, Karmaus W. Shift work and subfecundity: a European multicenter study. European Study Group on Infertility and Subfecundity. J Occup Environ Med. 1996;38(4):352–8.
27. Sheiner EK, Sheiner E, Carel R, Potashnik G, Shoham-Vardi I. Potential association between male infertility and occupational psychological stress. J Occup Environ Med. 2002;44(12):1093–9.
28. Tuntiseranee P, Olsen J, Geater A, Kor-anantakul O. Are long working hours and shiftwork risk factors for subfecundity? A study among couples from Southern Thailand. Occup Environ Med. 1998;55(2):99–105.
29. Irgens A, Kruger K, Ulstein M. The effect of male occupational exposure in infertile couples in Norway. J Occup Environ Med. 1999;41(12):1116–20.
30. Eisenberg ML, Chen Z, Ye A, Buck Louis GM. Relationship between physical occupational exposures and health on semen quality: data from the Longitudinal Investigation of Fertility and the Environment (LIFE) Study. Fertil Steril. 2015;103(5):1271–7. https://doi.org/10.1016/j.fertnstert.2015.02.010.
31. Pastuszak AW, Moon YM, Scovell J, Badal J, Lamb DJ, Link RE, et al. Poor sleep quality predicts hypogonadal symptoms and sexual dysfunction in male nonstandard shift workers. Urology. 2017;102:121–5. https://doi.org/10.1016/j.urology.2016.11.033.
32. Jensen MA, Hansen AM, Kristiansen J, Nabe-Nielsen K, Garde AH. Changes in the diurnal rhythms of cortisol, melatonin, and testosterone after 2, 4, and 7 consecutive night shifts in male police officers. Chronobiol Int. 2016;33(9):1–13. https://doi.org/10.1080/07420528.2016.1212869.
33. Smith AM, Morris P, Rowell KO, Clarke S, Jones TH, Channer KS. Junior doctors and the full shift rota – psychological and hormonal changes: a comparative cross-sectional study. Clin Med (Lond). 2006;6(2):174–7.
34. Touitou Y, Motohashi Y, Reinberg A, Touitou C, Bourdeleau P, Bogdan A, et al. Effect of shift work on the night-time secretory patterns of melatonin, prolactin, cortisol and testosterone. Eur J Appl Physiol Occup Physiol. 1990;60(4):288–92.
35. Papantoniou K, Pozo OJ, Espinosa A, Marcos J, Castano-Vinyals G, Basagana X, et al. Increased and mistimed sex hormone production in night shift workers. Cancer Epidemiol Biomark Prev. 2015;24(5):854–63. https://doi.org/10.1158/1055-9965.EPI-14-1271.
36. Axelsson J, Ingre M, Akerstedt T, Holmback U. Effects of acutely displaced sleep on testosterone. J Clin Endocrinol Metab. 2005;90(8):4530–5.
37. Bhasin S, Brito JP, Cunningham GR, Hayes FJ, Hodis HN, Matsumoto AM, et al. Testosterone therapy in men with hypogonadism: an Endocrine Society clinical practice guideline. J Clin Endocrinol Metab. 2018;103(5):1715–44. https://doi.org/10.1210/jc.2018-00229.
38. Peppard PE, Young T, Barnet JH, Palta M, Hagen EW, Hla KM. Increased prevalence of sleep-disordered breathing in adults. Am J Epidemiol. 2013;177(9):1006–14. https://doi.org/10.1093/aje/kws342.
39. Drager LF, McEvoy RD, Barbe F, Lorenzi-Filho G, Redline S, Initiative I. Sleep apnea and cardiovascular disease: lessons from recent trials and need for team science. Circulation. 2017;136(19):1840–50. https://doi.org/10.1161/CIRCULATIONAHA.117.029400.

40. Melehan KL, Hoyos CM, Hamilton GS, Wong KK, Yee BJ, McLachlan RI, et al. Randomised trial of CPAP and vardenafil on erectile and arterial function in men with obstructive sleep apnea and erectile dysfunction. J Clin Endocrinol Metab. 2018;103(4):1601–11. https://doi.org/10.1210/jc.2017-02389.
41. Torres M, Laguna-Barraza R, Dalmases M, Calle A, Pericuesta E, Montserrat JM, et al. Male fertility is reduced by chronic intermittent hypoxia mimicking sleep apnea in mice. Sleep. 2014;37(11):1757–65. https://doi.org/10.5665/sleep.4166.
42. Cignarelli A, Castellana M, Castellana G, Perrini S, Brescia F, Natalicchio A, et al. Effects of CPAP on testosterone levels in patients with obstructive sleep apnea: a meta-analysis study. Front Endocrinol (Lausanne). 2019;10:551. https://doi.org/10.3389/fendo.2019.00551.
43. Hoekema A, Stel AL, Stegenga B, van der Hoeven JH, Wijkstra PJ, van Driel MF, et al. Sexual function and obstructive sleep apnea-hypopnea: a randomized clinical trial evaluating the effects of oral-appliance and continuous positive airway pressure therapy. J Sex Med. 2007;4(4 Pt 2):1153–62.
44. Meston N, Davies RJ, Mullins R, Jenkinson C, Wass JA, Stradling JR. Endocrine effects of nasal continuous positive airway pressure in male patients with obstructive sleep apnoea. J Intern Med. 2003;254(5):447–54.
45. Luboshitzky R, Lavie L, Shen-Orr Z, Lavie P. Pituitary-gonadal function in men with obstructive sleep apnea. The effect of continuous positive airways pressure treatment. Neuroendocrinol Lett. 2003;24(6):463–7.
46. Santamaria JD, Prior JC, Fleetham JA. Reversible reproductive dysfunction in men with obstructive sleep apnea. Clin Endocrinol. 1988;28:461–70.
47. Liu PY, Yee BJ, Wishart SM, Jimenez M, Jung DG, Grunstein RR, et al. The short-term effects of high dose testosterone on sleep, breathing and function in older men. J Clin Endocrinol Metab. 2003;88(8):3605–13.
48. Schneider BK, Pickett CK, Zwillich CW, Weil JV, McDermott MT, Santen RJ, et al. Influence of testosterone on breathing during sleep. J Appl Physiol. 1986;61:618–23.
49. Snyder PJ, Peachey H, Hannoush P, Berlin JA, Loh L, Holmes JH, et al. Effect of testosterone treatment on bone mineral density in men over 65 years of age. J Clin Endocrinol Metab. 1999;84(6):1966–72.
50. Hoyos CM, Killick R, Yee BJ, Grunstein RR, Liu PY. Effects of testosterone therapy on sleep and breathing in obese men with severe obstructive sleep apnea: a randomised placebo-controlled trial. Clin Endocrinol. 2012;77:599–607. https://doi.org/10.1111/j.1365-2265.2012.04413.x.
51. Killick R, Wang D, Hoyos CM, Yee BJ, Grunstein RR, Liu PY. The effects of testosterone on ventilatory responses in men with obstructive sleep apnoea: a randomized placebo-controlled trial. J Sleep Res. 2013;22:331–6.
52. Matsumoto A, Sandblom RE, Schoene RB, Lee KA, Giblin EC, Pierson DJ, et al. Testosterone replacement in hypogonadal men: effects on obstructive sleep apnea, respiratory drives and sleep. Clin Endocrinol. 1985;22:713–21.
53. Calof OM, Singh AB, Lee ML, Kenny AM, Urban RJ, Tenover JL, et al. Adverse events associated with testosterone replacement in middle-aged and older men: a meta-analysis of randomized, placebo-controlled trials. J Gerontol A Biol Sci Med Sci. 2005;60(11):1451–7.

Chapter 6
Testosterone Therapy and Male Fertility

Robert E. Brannigan

6.1 Introduction

Testosterone is a pivotal hormone that is involved in the regulation of many facets of normal human physiology and function, including reproduction. Testosterone was first isolated by Dr. Ernst Laqueur in 1935, and it was approved for medical use 4 years later in 1939 [1]. However, it was not until approximately 70 years after its discovery that testosterone deficiency, as a medical condition, garnered increasing public awareness and overall visibility as a disorder whose treatment could benefit large numbers of aging males. These changes came mainly as exogenous testosterone was actively promoted as a therapy for men with both low serum testosterone levels and accompanying signs and symptoms of low testosterone, including decreased libido, erectile dysfunction, loss of energy, diminished mood, and sarcopenia. Increased public awareness of the links between low testosterone and numerous aging-related signs and symptoms coincided with a threefold increase in testosterone prescriptions for males over 40 years of age in the United States [2]. While many men benefitted from this therapy, some practitioners prescribed testosterone therapy to patients without performing a proper diagnostic workup (i.e., documenting a low serum testosterone level, determining that the patient had signs or symptoms of testosterone deficiency, etc.), without discussing the associated possible risks and benefits of therapy (i.e., suppression of spermatogenesis and infertility), and without providing appropriate longitudinal follow-up care. While testosterone therapy has provided substantial clinical benefits and relief from bothersome signs and symptoms associated with testosterone deficiency, these therapeutic gains do not come without potential downsides. As mentioned above, these drawbacks include impairment of male reproductive potential and resultant

R. E. Brannigan (✉)
Northwestern University, Feinberg School of Medicine, Evanston, IL, USA
e-mail: r-brannigan@northwestern.edu

© Springer Nature Switzerland AG 2021
J. P. Mulhall et al. (eds.), *Controversies in Testosterone Deficiency*,
https://doi.org/10.1007/978-3-030-77111-9_6

infertility, which can be either temporary or permanent. This chapter focuses on the important intersection between testosterone and male reproduction, including the unique therapeutic challenges encountered in treating males with testosterone deficiency who wish to preserve their future reproductive potential.

6.2 Male Reproduction

The hypothalamic-pituitary-gonadal (HPG) axis is a complex, highly integrated system that drives male reproductive processes at numerous levels, including central sexual desire, intratesticular spermatogenesis, and post-testicular accessory gland function. The endocrine initiation of male reproduction begins with the release of gonadotropin releasing hormone (GnRH) from the hypothalamus. GnRH is secreted from specialized neurons in the arcuate nucleus of the hypothalamus and is transported via the hypothalamic-pituitary portal microvascular system to the anterior pituitary gland. GnRH secretion occurs in a pulsatile fashion, with a rate of approximately 3.8 secretions every 6 hours appearing to be the optimal frequency for normal gonadal function. Abnormally increased or decreased frequency of secretory pulses can each result in disruption of the normal hormonal milieu [3]. In response to GnRH secretion, the anterior pituitary secretes the gonadotropins luteinizing hormone (LH) and follicle stimulating hormone (FSH). LH binds to the receptors of Leydig cells, stimulating testosterone production and secretion. FSH binds to the receptors of Sertoli cells and stimulates the translation of numerous proteins that support spermatogenesis. The HPG axis has several negative feedback loops, comprised predominately of estradiol and testosterone, which suppress the release of both LH and FSH from the anterior pituitary gland. In addition, inhibin B, a protein secreted by Sertoli cells, feeds back centrally and can inhibit pituitary FSH secretion without affecting LH secretion [3].

The testicle is encased within the tunica albuginea and comprises 250–300 distinct lobules. The testicular anatomy has classically been divided into three different compartments : the vascular, interstitial, and intraluminal compartments [4]. Each of these regions plays its own unique and important role in supporting spermatogenesis. The vascular compartment delivers the essential metabolic supplies to the testicle from the central circulation, including electrolytes, nutrients, fluid, and endocrine modulators. The testicular microvascular anatomy is characterized by capillaries that envelop but never penetrate the seminiferous tubules, a hallmark trait of the blood-testis barrier. The interstitial compartment is thus the proximate source of all fluid, nutrients, and electrolytes that facilitate the metabolic activities occurring within the seminiferous tubules. Additionally, Leydig cells secrete testosterone into the interstitial compartment fluid, where testosterone concentrations are on the order of 100–200 times higher than serum testosterone levels [5]. Collectively, the interstitial fluid compartment substances enter the intraluminal (seminiferous tubule) compartment via diffusion and/or active transport, where they stimulate and support Sertoli cell function and germ cell production. The intraluminal compartment – comprises the space within the seminiferous tubule – houses the Sertoli and germ cells and is the site of spermatogenesis. The Sertoli cells, which are directly regulated by testosterone, play a critical sustentacular role, providing both structural and functional support for spermatogenesis. The aforementioned blood-testis barrier is actually more aptly deemed a Sertoli cell barrier, composed of tight junctions, adherens junctions, and gap junctions between adjacent Sertoli cells. These structures subdivide the seminiferous tubule into a basal compartment that is exposed to blood and lymph fluid, and an adluminal compartment that is devoid of this exposure, thus shielding post-mitotic germ cells from the immune system. Sertoli cell protein products, including transferrin, clusterin, and insulin-like growth factor, all bind to germ cells and help regulate sperm production. Interestingly, the germ cells themselves are devoid of androgen receptors, and thus testosterone exerts only indirect effects on germ cell growth and development [6].

Spermatogenesis is a highly complex process that depends not only on systemic endocrine but also on local paracrine and autocrine mechanisms. While spermatogonia reside on the basement membrane, more mature and later stage germ cells, including primary spermatocytes, secondary spermatocytes, and spermatids, grow inward toward the lumen, filling the apical portion of the compartment. Spermatogenesis in humans follows a stratified and layered spiral configuration, with an intertwined, helical pattern along the length of the seminiferous tubule. In humans, the cycle of spermatogenesis from spermatogonial stage cell to ejaculated spermatozoon takes approximately 60–76 days, based on several kinetic studies performed using stable isotopes [7–9]. Once sperms exit the testicle, the excurrent ductal system (epididymis and vas deferens) and the male accessory glands (seminal vesicles and prostate gland), all androgen-dependent structures, facilitate sperm transport. Upon exiting the testicle via the efferent ductules, the sperm transit through the epididymis and ultimately, during seminal emission, through the vas deferens and ejaculatory duct. During seminal emission, the seminal vesicles and prostate gland also each respectively secrete fluid that proceeds into the prostatic urethra, and sperms expressed through the vas deferens and ejaculatory duct join this fluid collection to comprise the seminal clot. Shortly afterward, during sexual climax, the bladder neck closes, and the coordinated muscular contractions of the periurethral and pelvic muscles result in ejaculation. This event completes the process of sperm transport within the male, as the semen is propulsed through the urethra and out of the tip of the penis. All of these structures are, to varying degrees, dependent on androgens for their normal development and ongoing function.

6.3   Testosterone Deficiency and Male Infertility

Given the pivotal role that testosterone plays in establishing and maintaining normal male reproductive potential, the assessment of testosterone levels in men presenting for a fertility evaluation is a key aspect of the patient's diagnostic evaluation. According to the Practice Committee of the American Society for Reproductive

Medicine, an endocrine evaluation should be undertaken in infertile males who have at least one abnormal semen parameter, abnormal sexual function, or clinical findings that suggest the possible presence of an endocrinopathy. This endocrine evaluation should include, at a minimum, both serum FSH and testosterone levels as part of the initial endocrine workup [10]. Given the diurnal pattern of variation of testosterone secretion, with peak levels occurring soon after waking, a morning testosterone test time is generally recommended (unless the patient is sleeping during the day, in which case, the test should be obtained soon after waking) in order to avoid "false-positive" low levels, which can be seen in some men with afternoon or evening blood draws. If the initial serum testosterone level is low (<300 ng/dL), a repeat level is necessary in order to differentiate a truly low level from a sporadically low level. In addition to the above-mentioned diurnal secretory variation, low testosterone levels can also be reflective of the physiological variation in levels that occurs throughout the day and is linked to the pulsatile nature of GnRH, LH, and testosterone secretion. If the serum testosterone is low, the American Urological Association Guidelines on the Evaluation and Treatment of Testosterone Deficiency recommends that a serum LH level also be measured in order to determine if the patient suffers from secondary (hypogonadotropic) hypogonadism with a hypothalamic or pituitary defect versus primary (hypergonadotropic) hypogonadism with a primary testicular defect [11].

Patients with hypogonadotropic hypogonadism have low or normal serum LH levels, and adjunctive testing such as serum prolactin level, pituitary imaging, and iron studies is indicated in order to further investigate the underlying cause. Hypogonadotropic hypogonadism can result from abnormally low GnRH secretion by the hypothalamus, a condition that can either be congenital, as in the case of Kallmann syndrome, or acquired, resulting from injury or damage to the hypothalamus. Similarly, hypogonadotropic hypogonadism can result from pituitary abnormalities, including prolactinomas, infiltrating brain tumors, trauma, and iatrogenic injury from surgery or radiation therapy. A pituitary MRI should be considered in the setting of unexplained low LH and FSH levels, especially when the serum testosterone is <150 ng/dL. This pituitary imaging can help to identify sellar lesions, including pituitary adenomas, prolactinomas, infiltrative processes, or parasellar conditions [11]. Patients with hypogonadotropic hypogonadism typically have decreased or altogether absent spermatogenesis due to their abnormally low testosterone and FSH levels.

Patients with hypergonadotropic hypogonadism have elevated serum LH +/− FSH levels and low serum testosterone levels. The primary issue in these patients is an intrinsic testicular abnormality, with diminished testosterone production. When these findings are unexplained, and particularly in cases of azoospermia, adjunctive testing could include chromosome analysis to evaluate for conditions such as Klinefelter syndrome (47, XXY karyotype), which occurs in approximately 1:500 men [11].

6.4   Adverse Effects of Exogenous Androgens and Spermatogenesis

Exogenous androgens can have profound inhibitory effects on spermatogenesis. As detailed earlier, administration of exogenous androgens results in the suppression of LH and FSH secretion via the negative feedback loop that is an essential aspect of HPG axis self-regulation.

The adverse effects of androgens on spermatogenesis have been best studied in numerous male contraception studies with testosterone administered as the contraceptive agent. Most of these studies utilized subjects who started with baseline normal serum testosterone levels, and most study subjects recovered normal levels of spermatogenesis after cessation of the testosterone. An integrated study by Liu et al. combined data from 30 contraception studies involving 1549 healthy men who were started on exogenous testosterone to determine contraceptive effects [12]. The authors found that recovery of spermatogenesis to normal sperm concentrations (>20 million sperm/mL) occurred within 6 months of testosterone cessation in 67% of study subjects, within 1 year in 90%, within 16 months in 96%, and finally within 2 years in 100% of subjects. It is very important to stress, though, that these study subjects were normal men with normal baseline testosterone levels and semen analyses. Neither men with testosterone deficiency nor men with infertility were considered in this study. Samplaski ct al. assessed 59 subjects who presented with complaints of infertility while on exogenous testosterone [13]. The authors found that 88.4% of these infertile study subjects were azoospermic while on testosterone, and by 6 months after testosterone cessation, 65% of the patients who had no other identifiable cause for azoospermia had recovered spermatogenesis. In this retrospective study, there was no set regimen regarding the medical approach to treating testosterone deficiency once the testosterone was halted, and some of the patients were on various combinations of agents including clomiphene citrate, human chorionic gonadotropin (hCG), anastrozole, and/or menotropin. Kohn et al. studied 66 males who presented for an infertility workup, were on exogenous testosterone therapy, and were found to have a sperm concentration of ≤1 million sperm/mL. In this study, the authors aimed to determine the recovery of spermatogenesis with initiation of hCG therapy after cessation of exogenous testosterone. The authors set a total motile sperm count (TMSC) of 5 million as an indicator of recovery of spermatogenesis. The authors found that 65% of the patients presenting with azoospermia and 92% of the patients presenting with cryptozoospermia achieved a TMSC of 5 million with this regimen. An important consideration for this study and similar studies is that baseline semen testing before initiation of exogenous testosterone is missing on the majority of subjects [14].

6.5 Alternative Therapies for the Treatment of Testosterone Deficiency

The American Urological Association Guidelines on the Evaluation and Treatment of Testosterone Deficiency recommends that clinicians may use "alternative therapies" alone or in combination when treating men with testosterone deficiency who desire to maintain their fertility. These alternative therapies include hCG, selective estrogen receptor modulators (SERMs), and aromatase inhibitors alone or in combination with one another. This is particularly relevant, given the high prevalence of males presenting for a fertility evaluation who have nonobstructive azoospermia of oligospermia. More specifically, 15% of couples experience infertility, and among them, approximately half will have a male factor involved. Given the inhibitory effects of exogenous testosterone on intratesticular testosterone production and spermatogenesis, these alternative therapies offer a critically important pathway to optimize endogenous testosterone production and improve the signs and symptoms associated with testosterone deficiency, including infertility. While these alternative therapies each have different mechanisms of action, they share the same common end result of optimizing endogenous testosterone production. Among these alternative therapies, only hCG has been approved for use in males, with an indication only in treating hypogonadotropic hypogonadism. At the current time, there are a limited number of studies detailing the effects of these agents on male reproductive potential, and the quality of these studies in aggregate is highly variable. Despite the paucity of data on the use of these agents, there are several noteworthy studies that provide important insights into these medications, and they can serve as a useful guide for clinicians who consider prescribing these medications for patients, as detailed below.

6.5.1 Aromatase Inhibitors

Aromatase inhibitors block the conversion of testosterone to estradiol, and in doing this, they diminish the depletion of testosterone that occurs during this conversion. The resultant decrease in estradiol levels caused by aromatase inhibition also results in less estradiol negative feedback centrally on the HPG axis. The end result is increased LH secretion and an increase in testosterone secretion.

Pavlovich et al. described a specific "treatable endocrinopathy" within infertile males, consisting of low testosterone, elevated estradiol, and an abnormally low testosterone: estradiol ratio (<10:1) [15]. Two separate studies assessed the effects of treating this condition with aromatase inhibitors, and the authors found that oligospermic subjects experienced an increase in T:E ratio as well as an increase in semen parameters [15, 16]. A subsequent study at the same institution found that aromatase inhibitor therapy used in men who had azoospermia, a serum testosterone level <300 ng/dL, and a T:E ratio <10:1 resulted in no increase in rates of sperm retrieval, pregnancy, or live birth when compared to men not on this therapy. Finally, Ramasamy et al. reported on a series of azoospermic males with Klinefelter syndrome who were treated with alternative therapies (aromatase inhibitors, hCG, SERMS), either alone or in various combinations [17]. Results demonstrated improved sperm retrieval rates among those who experienced increased T:E ratios and T levels >250 ng/dl, suggesting a possible role for these agents in this clinical setting.

Anastrozole is an aromatase inhibitor with good clinical efficacy, and it is commonly used at dosages in males ranging from 0.05 to 1 mg every 1–3 days. Anastrozole's t_{max} (time to reach maximal serum concentration) is 2–5 hours, and the $t_{1/2}$ (half-life) is 40–50 hours [11]. Side effects are generally mild and well tolerated, but can include nausea, hot flashes, hypertension, back pain, bone pain, dyspnea, and peripheral edema. The oral route of administration is convenient for patients, avoiding potential barriers sometimes seen with injectable agents.

When prescribing aromatase inhibitors, several important caveats should be followed. First, aromatase inhibitors should in general not be used for long durations of time because of potential deceases in bone mineral density that can occur with suppression of estradiol [18]. However, with regular, periodic follow-up and careful management of aromatase inhibitor dosing, estradiol can be maintained within the normal range, which will minimize the potential risk of bone density loss [11]. Finally, in those patients for whom aromatase inhibition results in persistently elevated estradiol levels, the therapy should be stopped due to lack of efficacy [11].

6.5.2   Human Chorionic Gonadotropin (hCG)

Human chorionic gonadotropin is an LH agonist that is approved by FDA for use in treating men with hypogonadotropic hypogonadism. The bulk of the existing medical literature regarding this agent has been conducted in men with congenital (idiopathic) hypogonadotropic hypogonadism [19, 20]. There are fewer studies characterizing the use of hCG in the broader population of adult males with testosterone deficiency not stemming from primary pituitary dysfunction. Nonetheless, several publications provide valuable information for clinicians considering the use of hCG in this wider context. Liu et al. evaluated the effects of hCG in a cohort of older men with a mean age of 67 years and androgen deficiency [21]. This study was a double-blind, placebo-controlled, randomized trial, and when compared to patients receiving placebo, those patients receiving hCG had an approximately 150% increase in their serum total testosterone level. The authors concluded that aging males enjoy some level of "testicular responsiveness" to hCG therapy. Some investigators have described the use of hCG concurrently with exogenous testosterone therapy in an effort to maintain intratesticular testosterone production, with putative advantages including the maintenance of spermatogenesis. Coviello et al. reported that co-administration of low-dose hCG with exogenous testosterone maintained intratesticular testosterone production [22]. In their cohort, the authors found that exogenous intramuscular testosterone therapy suppressed intratesticular testosterone levels 94% from baseline. Subsequently, when hCG 250 IU every other day was added to the regimen, intratesticular testosterone levels were only 7% less than baseline, and when hCG 500 IU every other day was added to the regimen, intratesticular testosterone levels rose to 26% above the baseline level. Hsieh et al. subsequently found that in a cohort of 26 men treated with hCG 500 IU every other day combined with either daily topical testosterone gel or weekly intramuscular testosterone, no patients became azoospermic. Furthermore, no changes in semen parameters were observed over the 12-month follow-up period, and 9/26 patients achieved a pregnancy with their partner during the study interval [23]. These publications collectively suggest that hCG given concurrently with exogenous testosterone can preserve both intratesticular testosterone production and fertility for men on exogenous testosterone therapy.

hCG is commonly used as monotherapy in males at dosages ranging from 500 to 4000 IU subcutaneously or intramuscularly 2–3 times per week. hCG's t_{max} is 12 hours and the $t_{1/2}$ is 2 days [11]. Side effects are typically mild and can include headache, irritability, depression, fatigue, edema, gynecomastia, and injection site pain [11]. The injection route of administration is less convenient than oral forms of alternative therapies, but this downside is often offset by the direct, LH-agonist mechanism of action.

6.5.3   Selective Estrogen Receptor Modulators (SERMs)

Selective estrogen receptor modulators are oral agents that block estradiol negative feedback centrally, resulting in an increase in LH secretion. Among the three classes of alternative therapies, SERMs are the most well studied in terms of putative fertility preservation benefits. Several reports reveal favorable clinical response, with serum testosterone level increases mirroring those seen for patients on testosterone gel therapy [24]. Clomiphene citrate, the most commonly used SERM in the setting of male hypogonadism, has been shown to be less expensive than testosterone gel therapy and also to be very well tolerated in terms of its side effect profile [11]. Two randomized, controlled trials found that for men with testosterone deficiency, treatment with SERMs resulted in stable sperm concentrations, whereas treatment with exogenous testosterone resulted in significantly decreased parameters [25, 26]. In a prospective, double-blind, randomized, controlled trial, Helo et al. found that clomiphene citrate therapy led to significantly higher serum testosterone levels when compared to anastrozole therapy [27]. Alternatively, anastrozole led to significantly higher T:E ratios than did clomiphene citrate. In the end, neither therapeutic approach led to significant changes in semen parameters among patients within the cohort.

Clomiphene citrate is commonly prescribed at dosages ranging from 25 to 50 mg every 1–2 days. Clomiphene's t_{max} is 5 hours and the $t_{1/2}$ is 5–7 days [11]. Side effects are typically mild and can include headache, visual symptoms, and flushing. The oral route of administration is a substantial advantage when compared to non-oral forms of alternative therapies.

When prescribing SERMs, several important points should be kept in mind. First, a serum LH level should be obtained after starting therapy. If the LH level remains abnormally low in the setting of a persistently low testosterone level, then an increase in the dosage of the SERM can be considered [11]. This maneuver sometimes results in further optimization of testosterone levels. However, if after initiating the SERM, the serum testosterone level remains low in the setting of an elevated LH level, then dose escalation of the SERM is not likely to result in additional increases in the serum testosterone level, as the primary issue is likely testicular failure [11]. The use of SERMS also results in a paradoxical decline in semen parameters in an estimated 17–24% of men, although the exact rate and etiology for these findings are understudied [28]. Given these observations, routine monitoring of semen parameters is warranted among men treated with SERMs who wish to maintain fertility.

6.6 Treatment of Testosterone Deficiency in "Special Populations"

Several "special populations" of patients warrant consideration in this chapter. Each patient group has unique challenges in the management of their testosterone deficiency, and as a result, up-front discussions with these patients are important in order to clarify their expectations and convey a clear sense of likely outcomes related to therapeutic intervention.

6.6.1 The Aging Male

Aging males often pursue testosterone therapy in an effort to offset numerous aging-related changes, including physical, cognitive, and sexual signs and symptoms. Credible literature supports the benefits of testosterone replacement therapy in improving erectile dysfunction, low libido, low bone mineral density, decreased lean body mass, and depressive symptoms related to low testosterone [11]. However, the literature at this time is inconclusive regarding testosterone's benefits in improving fatigue/low energy, decreased cognitive function, dyslipidemia, measures of metabolic abnormalities related to diabetes mellitus, and quality of life [11].

Some clinicians make broad assumptions about patients and their desires for future fertility based upon traits such as a patient's age, existing number of children, sexual orientation, and marital status. Unfortunately, these assumptions are often incorrect and may result in a clinician initiating exogenous testosterone with its resultant contraceptive effects in a man who desires future children. The American Urological Association's guideline document on the Evaluation and Management of Testosterone Deficiency strongly recommends that exogenous testosterone should not be prescribed to men who are currently trying to conceive, given the commonly seen resultant suppression of the HPG axis and spermatogenesis. Even if a patient reports no interest in current or near-term conception, they should be made aware of the contraceptive effects of androgen therapy. Some of these men might change their mind in the future, and they should be made aware of the process of stopping exogenous testosterone and possibly converting to one of the above-mentioned alternative therapeutic regimens.

6.6.2   The Male Who Abuses Anabolic Steroids

The first reports of abuse of androgens occurred during the 1954 Olympics, when Russian weightlifters were given exogenous testosterone in order to increase strength and performance [29]. Anabolic steroid abuse increased significantly within the general population in the 1980s, with abusers looking to enhance appearance and/or improve athletic performance. In 1990, the US Congress passed the Anabolic Steroid Control Act, providing definitions for these agents and subjecting them to federal control. Shortly thereafter, illicit labs and medical tourism increased, as abusers sought avenues around these legal restrictions. The end result has been the emergence of a sophisticated "underground marketplace" and culture where patients acquire and self-treat with these illicit agents [30]. Over the long term, despite efforts at "cycling" and "stacking" agents on their regimen, these patients often suffer from chronic suppression of the HPG axis, progressive testicular atrophy, and azoospermia [31]. This condition, deemed "anabolic steroid induced hypogonadism" (ASIH), can be extremely challenging for clinicians to effectively treat. While most cases of ASIH-related azoospermia will resolve spontaneously within 4–12 months, some patients experience persistent oligo- or azoospermia. Rahnema et al. have described a treatment algorithm for symptomatic ASIH that combines a graduated tapering of the anabolic steroid over time with initiation of alternative therapies such as SERMs and, if needed, hCG [30]. The end aim is to drive up endogenous testosterone production, which might not only treat more generalized symptoms but also improve spermatogenesis and fertility potential. For those patients who remain persistently azoospermic despite these therapeutic maneuvers, microdissection testicular sperm extraction ("micro-TESE") is an option, although no large data sets exist regarding this patient population's clinical outcomes, including sperm retrieval, pregnancy, and live birth rates.

6.6.3   The Male with Hypogonadotropic Hypogonadism

Hypogonadotropic hypogonadism can be either a congenital or an acquired condition. Congenital hypogonadotropic hypogonadism (CHH) typically results from a genetic deficiency of GnRH secretion, and to date over 30 etiologic mutations have been described [32]. Patients typically present with lack of pubertal development, prompting a medical workup and diagnosis.

Acquired hypogonadotropic hypogonadism can arise due to infiltrating or impinging tumors, trauma, and iatrogenic causes such as surgery and radiation therapy. If the condition onsets prior to adolescence, patients will typically present with failure to initiate puberty. For those patients in whom the onset is post-pubertal, signs and symptoms of testosterone deficiency can develop, including regression of secondary sexual characteristic, loss of libido, erectile dysfunction, and infertility.

Therapies for these patients consist of replacing the deficient gonadotropins, namely using hCG, and, if FSH is abnormally low, recombinant FSH (r-FSH). While these therapies are usually effective, clinical utilization is often limited by the high cost of medication and necessity for self-injection. These issues include the cost of gonadotropin therapy and subcutaneous or intramuscular route of administration.

6.6.4   The Male with Klinefelter Syndrome

Klinefelter syndrome (47, XXY) is a congenital form of hypergonadotropic hypogonadism and accounts for approximately two-thirds of chromosomal abnormalities among infertile men. This condition has a high prevalence, affecting 1:500 males. Klinefelter syndrome is also associated with numerous congenital abnormalities of the testicle, including atrophy, fibrosis, and decreased or altogether absent spermatogenesis. These patients typically have azoospermia, but despite this azoospermia, over half will have active spermatogenesis occurring within the testicle. Several studies have assessed the role of hormonal optimization within these patients prior to micro-TESE, with varying results [33, 34]. While there is no favored regimen at this time, key findings in the literature for this patient population include optimizing the T:E ratio > 10:1, commonly through the use of aromatase inhibitors, and concurrent optimization of testosterone >300 ng/dL via the use of hCG and/or SERMs. The Cornell group reports a 65% sperm retrieval rate for their series of patients with Klinefelter syndrome, with overall favorable pregnancy rates of 40% [34]. Keys to success in treating these patients include a runup of hormonal optimization of at least 3 months duration prior to the micro-TESE and careful consideration of the use of an aromatase inhibitor as part of the treatment regimen, given the high prevalence of obesity with associated abnormally high serum estradiol levels. While these patients have a 47, XXY karyotype, their gametes are typically euploid, with only a single X or Y sex chromosome. Klinefelter syndrome is a unique chromosomal condition in this way, as it is very rare for a patient with Klinefelter syndrome to father an offspring with the same abnormal karyotype. Most offspring are, in fact, euploid (46, XX or XY).

6.7 Conclusions

Testosterone deficiency is a highly prevalent condition affecting large numbers of males. Exogenous testosterone formulations are the most widely used forms of therapy for affected patients, but these agents commonly cause suppression of endogenous testosterone production and result in impaired spermatogenesis. "Alternative therapies," as described in the 2018 American Urological Association Guidelines on the Evaluation and Treatment of Testosterone Deficiency, each work via different mechanisms but share the common end result of improving endogenous testosterone production. Furthermore, as a result of the increased endogenous testosterone, these agents also often improve spermatogenesis and thus enhance male fertility potential. Clinicians should thus become both familiar and comfortable with the use of alternative therapies in patients desiring treatment of their testosterone deficiency with concurrent fertility preservation.

References

1. Nieschlag E, Nieschlag S. Endocrine history: the history of discovery, synthesis and development of testosterone for clinical use. Eur J Endocrinol. 2019;180(6):R201–12.
2. Baillargeon J, Urban RJ, Ottenbacher KJ, Pierson KS, Goodwin JS. Trends in androgen prescribing in the United States, 2001 to 2011. JAMA Intern Med. 2013;173(15):1465–6.
3. Plymate SR. Hypogonadism in men: an overview. In: Bagatell CJ, Bremner WJ, editors. Androgens in health and disease. Totowa: Humana Press Inc.; 2003. p. 45–88.
4. Liu PY, Veldhuis JD. Hypothalamo-pituitary unit, testis, and male accessory organs. In: Strauss III JF, Barbieri RL, Gargiulo AR, editors. Yen and Jaffe's reproductive endocrinology: physiology, pathophysiology, and clinical management. 8th ed. Philadelphia: Elsevier, Inc.; 2019. p. 285–300.
5. Hinton BT, Turner TT. The seminiferous tubular microenvironment. In: Desjardins C, Ewing LL, editors. Cell and molecular biology of the testis. New York: Oxford University Press; 1993. p. 238–65.
6. Suárez-Quian CA, Martínez-García F, Nistal M, Regadera J. Androgen receptor distribution in adult human testis. J Clin Endocrinol Metab. 1999;84(1):350–8.
7. Clermont Y. Kinetics of spermatogenesis in mammals: seminiferous epithelium cycle and spermatogonial renewal. Physiol Rev. 1972;52(1):198–236.
8. Heller CH, Clermont Y. Kinetics of the germinal epithelium in man. Recent Prog Horm Res. 1964;20:545–75.

9. Misell LM, Holochwost D, Boban D, Santi N, Shefi S, Hellerstein MK, Turek PJ. A stable isotope-mass spectrometric method for measuring human spermatogenesis kinetics in vivo. J Urol. 2006;175(1):242–6.
10. Practice Committee of the American Society for Reproductive Medicine. Diagnostic evaluation of the infertile male: a committee opinion. Fertil Steril. 2015;103(3):e18–25.
11. Mulhall JP, Trost LW, Brannigan RE, Kurtz EG, Redmon JB, Chiles KA, Lightner DJ, Miner MM, Murad MH, Nelson CJ, Platz EA, Ramanathan LV, Lewis RW. Evaluation and management of testosterone deficiency: AUA guideline. J Urol. 2018;200(2):423–32.
12. Liu PY, Swerdloff RS, Anawalt BD, et al. Determinants of the rate and extent of spermatogenic suppression during hormonal male contraception: an integrated analysis. J Clin Endocrinol Metab. 2008;93:1774.
13. Samplaski MK, Loai Y, Wong K, et al. Testosterone use in the male infertility population: prescribing patterns and effects on semen and hormonal parameters. Fertil Steril. 2014;101:64.
14. Kohn TP, Louis MR, Pickett SM, et al. Age and duration of testosterone therapy predict time to return of sperm count after human chorionic gonadotropin therapy. Fertil Steril. 2017;107:351.
15. Pavlovich CP, King P, Goldstein M, et al. Evidence of a treatable endocrinopathy in infertile men. J Urol. 2001;165:837.
16. Raman JD, Schlegel PN. Aromatase inhibitors for male infertility. J Urol. 2002;167:624.
17. Ramasamy R, Ricci JA, Palermo GD, et al. Successful fertility treatment for Klinefelter's Syndrome. J Urol. 2009;182:1108.
18. Burnett-Bowie SA, McKay EA, Lee H, et al. Effects of aromatase inhibition on bone mineral density and bone turnover in older men with low testosterone levels. J Clin Endocrinol Metab. 2009;94:4785.
19. Bistritzer T, Lunenfeld B, Passwell JH, et al. Hormonal therapy and pubertal development in boys with selective hypogonadotropic hypogonadism. Fertil Steril. 1989;52:302.
20. Vicari E, Mongioi A, Calogero AE, et al. Therapy with human chorionic gonadotrophin alone induces spermatogenesis in men with isolated hypogonadotrophic hypogonadism--long-term follow-up. Int J Androl. 1992;15:320.
21. Liu PY, Wishart SM, Handelsman DJ. A double-blind, placebo-controlled, randomized clinical trial of recombinant human chorionic gonadotropin on muscle strength and physical function and activity in older men with partial age-related androgen deficiency. J Clin Endocrinol Metab. 2002;87:3125.
22. Coviello AD, Matsumoto AM, Bremner WJ, et al. Low-dose human chorionic gonadotropin maintains intratesticular testosterone in normal men with testosterone-induced gonadotropin suppression. J Clin Endocrinol Metab. 2005;90:2595–602.
23. Hsieh TC, Pastuszak AW, Hwang K, et al. Concomitant intramuscular human chorionic gonadotropin preserves spermatogenesis in men undergoing testosterone replacement therapy. J Urol. 2013;189:647.
24. Taylor F, Levine L. Clomiphene citrate and testosterone gel replacement therapy for male hypogonadism: efficacy and treatment cost. J Sex Med. 2010;7:269.
25. Kim ED, McCullough A, Kaminetsky J. Oral enclomiphene citrate raises testosterone and preserves sperm counts in obese hypogonadal men, unlike topical testosterone: restoration instead of replacement. BJU Int. 2016;117:677.
26. Wiehle RD, Fontenot GK, Wike J, et al. Enclomiphene citrate stimulates testosterone production while preventing oligospermia: a randomized phase II clinical trial comparing topical testosterone. Fertil Steril. 2014;102:720.
27. Helo S, Ellen J, Mechlin C, et al. A randomized prospective double-blind comparison trial of clomiphene citrate and anastrozole in raising testosterone in hypogonadal infertile men. J Sex Med. 2015;12:1761.
28. Gundewar T, Kuchakulla M, Ramasamy R. A paradoxical decline in semen parameters in men treated with clomiphene citrate: a systematic review. Andrologia. 2020;27:e13848. Epub ahead of print.

29. Wade N. Anabolic steroids: doctors denounce them, but athletes aren't listening. Science. 1972;176(4042):1399–403.
30. Fink J, Schoenfeld BJ, Hackney AC, et al. Anabolic-androgenic steroids: procurement and administration practices of doping athletes. Phys Sportsmed. 2019;47(1):10–4.
31. Rahnema CD, Lipshultz LI, Crosnoe LE, Kovac JR, Kim ED. Anabolic steroid-induced hypogonadism: diagnosis and treatment. Fertil Steril. 2014;101(5):1271–9.
32. Young J, Xu C, Papadakis GE, et al. Clinical management of congenital hypogonadotropic hypogonadism. Endocr Rev. 2019;40(2):669–710.
33. Fainberg J, Hayden RP, Schlegel PN. Fertility management of Klinefelter syndrome. Expert Rev Endocrinol Metab. 2019;14(6):369–80.
34. Dabaja AA, Schlegel PN. Microdissection testicular sperm extraction: an update. Asian J Androl. 2013;15(1):35–9.

Chapter 7
Testosterone and Prostate Effects

Carolyn A. Salter and John P. Mulhall

7.1 Introduction

Historically, testosterone (T) was thought to be involved in negative prostate events such as the growth of benign or malignant prostate tissue. This notion stems from the seminal 1941 article by Huggins and Hodges, which demonstrated that in men with metastatic prostate cancer (CaP), surgical castration led to a reduction in acid phosphatase levels, while administration of exogenous T led to an increase in these levels [1]. Our understanding has been further expanded with the concept of the saturation model, which suggests that above a certain T threshold, the androgen receptors are maximally stimulated and, thus, further increases in T levels have no additional effects on prostate cells [2]. However, at lower levels of T, prostate cells do respond to increased T levels, and changes in prostate tissue may occur. While the exact T saturation threshold in humans is not known, animal studies suggest that this is near-castrate levels and is at sub-physiologic levels in humans [2]. More recent data suggests that this total testosterone (TT) threshold is <250 ng/dL (8.67 nmol/L), although there is interindividual variability [3]. This chapter focuses on the effects of T on prostate tissues.

7.2 Prostate-Specific Antigen (PSA) Changes

Data from the Testim Registry in the US (TRiUS) nicely demonstrates the effect of T on PSA levels. This registry contains data of 451 men with testosterone deficiency (TD). These men were separated into two groups: those with TT < 250 ng/dL

C. A. Salter (✉) · J. P. Mulhall
Department of Urology, Memorial Sloan Kettering Cancer Center, New York, NY, USA
e-mail: mulhalj1@mskcc.org

© Springer Nature Switzerland AG 2021
J. P. Mulhall et al. (eds.), *Controversies in Testosterone Deficiency*,
https://doi.org/10.1007/978-3-030-77111-9_7

(8.67 nmol/L) (n = 197) and those with TT ≥ 250 ng/dL (8.67 nmol/L) (n = 254) [4]. At lower levels of TT, i.e., TT < 250 ng/dL (8.67 nmol/L), TT was loosely correlated with PSA (r = 0.20, p = 0.005) as was free T (FT), r = 0.22, p = 0.03. In contrast, this correlation was not seen in men with TT ≥ 250 ng/dL (8.67 nmol/L) [4]. These men were then evaluated after 12 months of T therapy (TTH). Results showed statistically significant PSA changes in men with TT < 250 ng/dL (8.67 nmol/L), with a mean increase in PSA of 0.19 ± 0.61 ng/mL (21.9%, p = 0.02). Those with baseline TT ≥250 ng/dL (8.67 nmol/L) experienced similar increases, although these were not statistically significant (0.28 ± 1.18 ng/mL, or 14.1%, p = 0.06). The highest observed PSA was within the first month of TTH followed by subsequent decline [4].

Marks et al. [5], evaluated 40 men with TD, as defined by symptoms and TT < 300 ng/dL (10.40 nmol/L). Men were randomized to intramuscular T (IMT) or placebo and were evaluated (to include prostate biopsies) at baseline and at 6 months [5]. The primary endpoint was intraprostatic T or dihydrotestosterone (DHT) levels, which were unchanged in the TTH group between baseline and 6 months (p = 0.29 and 0.51, respectively). However, PSA was higher after 6 months of TTH: 2.29 ng/mL (IQR 0.40–7.19) versus 1.55 ng/mL (IQR 0.30–5.80), p < 0.001 [5]. Similarly, when comparing the change in PSA between TTH and placebo, results were higher among TTH men at 0.90 ± 0.89 ng/mL versus 0.60 ± 1.55 ng/mL, p = 0.008.

Snyder et al. [6] evaluated 790 men ≥65 years old with TD, defined as TT < 275 ng/dL (9.53 nmol/L). Men were randomized 1:1 to T gel versus placebo for 1 year. At the completion of therapy, 23 TTH men were found to have PSA rises of >1 ng/ml compared to 8 in placebo (no p-value; study not specifically designed to compare adverse events between cohorts) [6].

Calof et al. [7] conducted a meta-analysis of 19 double-blinded placebo-controlled TTH trials with a total of 651 men on TTH and 433 on placebo. All studies included men ≥45 years old who were on TTH ≥ 90 days [7]. Results showed that "prostate events" as a whole were higher in the TTH group (OR 1.78, 95% CI 1.07–2.95). However, differences with individual prostate events, including PSA changes, were not statistically significant between the two groups. Specifically, PSA increases of >1.5 ng/mL or total PSA > 4 ng/dL occurred in 41.6 per 1000 patient-years in the placebo group versus 57.1 in the TTH group, OR 1.19 (95% CI 0.67–2.09) [7].

Arguably the strongest data on the role of TTH in PSA changes comes from the supporting text of the American Urological Association (AUA) Testosterone Deficiency guidelines [8]. A meta-analysis was performed on nine randomized control trials with a total of 2601 men. All trials compared TTH versus placebo in men with baseline TT < 350 ng/dL (12.14 nmol/L). The meta-analysis demonstrated findings that were borderline (but not statistically) significant for a mildly elevated PSA (OR 1.71, 95% CI 0.98–3.00; note that CI >1.00 is required for significance) [8].

In summary, the above data are inconclusive and somewhat contradictory. Results seem to suggest a possible effect of TTH on increasing PSA, although the overall effect is likely minor and appears to be more prominent among men with lower baseline TT levels. Larger, adequately powered series dedicated to specifically evaluating changes in PSA are required to definitively address whether TTH truly increases PSA, particularly in men with normal baseline TT levels.

7.3 Prostate Volume Changes

In Marks et al.'s [5] study of men on TTH versus placebo for 6 months, there was no change in prostate volume as measured by MRI (magnetic resonance imaging). This held true for total prostate volume [43.8 (15.5–112.0) versus 42.0 (19.8–117.9) mL; $p = 0.16$] and for the volume of the transition zone [21.8 (4.8–76.5) versus 15.4 (4.1–47.8) mL; $p = 0.58$] [5].

Liu et al. [9] also evaluated the effect of T levels on prostate volume. They evaluated 148 men aged ≥45 years old as part of a free health screening. The men underwent a transrectal ultrasound, completed the International Prostate Symptom Score (IPSS), and had PSA and T labs completed [9]. Their mean age was 59.8 years with a mean TT of 488 ± 170 ng/dL (16.64 ± 5.89 nmol/L) and FT of 8.4 ± 2.8 ng/dL (0.29 ± 0.10 nmol/L) . Results demonstrated that T did not correlate with prostate volume ($p = 0.35$ for TT and 0.45 for FT, respectively). On multivariable analysis (MVA) of predictors of prostate volume, only age was a significant predictor ($p < 0.001$) [9]. This provides further evidence that T levels do not influence prostate volume. However, it is important to note that these men had normal T levels and only a minority of patients had T levels close to the previously described saturation point.

In contrast to the above studies, Behre et al. [10] performed a study evaluating prostate volumes among men with much lower TT levels. Specifically, the authors compared 47 men with untreated TD, 78 men with TD on TTH for ≥6 months, and 75 men with normal TT levels [10]. The mean TT level for the TD group was 150 ng/dL (5.2 nmol/L) (95% CI 127–173) compared to 554 ng/dL (19.21 nmol/L) (95% CI 494–611) and 577 ng/dL (20.01 nmol/L) (95% CI 539–614) for TD on TTH and normal TT groups, respectively. Baseline prostate volumes were much lower in the TD groups at 12.2 mL (95% CI 11.0–13.5) compared to 21.3 mL (95% CI 19.9–22.8) in the TD on TTH and 22.9 mL (95% CI 21.4–24.4) in the normal T group, $p < 0.05$ [10]. A multivariable analysis of predictors of prostate volume was performed separately for each of the three patient groups. Interestingly, TT levels were only significantly associated with prostate volume in the TD group ($p = 0.006$) [10]. These findings are consistent with the previously described saturation model, in that, at lower baseline TT levels (i.e., below the saturation point), increases in TT result in concomitant increases in prostate volume.

7.4   Lower Urinary Tract Symptoms (LUTS)

LUTS can be measured subjectively, usually using a validated questionnaire called the IPSS (International Prostate Symptom Score), or objectively using a uroflow rate, which measures the strength of the urinary stream. The IPSS is adapted from the AUA Symptom Index for Benign Prostatic Hyperplasia [11] and includes seven questions for symptoms such as weak or intermittent urinary stream, frequency, urgency, and straining to urinate as well as a question on quality of life. Higher scores denote more severe symptoms. Marks et al. [5] evaluated LUTS in men after 6 months of TTH or placebo. After 6 months of TTH, when compared to baseline values, there was no change in IPSS score (13.0 [IQR 0–26.0] to 12.5 [0–30], $p = 0.43$ or with uroflow rates (14.0 [IQR 4.0–31.0] to 10.6 [IQR 4.8 to 18.9] mL/sec, $p = 0.09$ [5]. Similarly, when compared to the placebo group, there were no differences in IPSS score (+1.43 ± 8.14 versus −1.21 ± 7.74, $p = 0.30$) or uroflow rates (−3.66 ± 7.48 versus −3.44 ± 7.27 mL/sec, $p = 0.94$) among the men treated with TTH [5].

Snyder et al. [6] also demonstrated no change in LUTS based on IPSS score in men on TTH versus placebo. After 1 year of treatment, the rate of men with moderately severe LUTS (as determined by an IPSS score > 19) was similar in TTH and placebo groups (27 versus 26 men, respectively; no p-value provided) [6]. Similarly, Liu et al. [9] in their evaluation of the impact of T levels on prostate parameters found that neither TT nor FT was correlated with IPSS scores ($p = 0.26$ for TT and 0.74 for FT) [9]. In Behre et al.'s [10] study that compared prostate volume in men with untreated TD, TD on TTH for ≥6 months, and normal T, uroflow was also compared, with no differences observed among cohorts [10]. Thus, these studies all suggest no role of T in LUTS.

While the Calof et al.'s meta-analysis noted a higher rate of prostate events in the TTH men overall (OR 1.78, 95% CI 1.07–2.95), this did not hold true when evaluating specific prostate events [7]. For example, IPSS increases were similar (2.8 per 1000 patient-years in placebo versus 5.5 in TTH, OR 1.08 (95% CI 0.46–2.52). Episodes of acute urinary retention were also equivalent (0 in placebo versus 2.2 per 1000 patient-years in TTH group, OR 0.99, 95% CI 0.40–2.44) [7]. It is thought that this can be explained by the fact that statistically these calculations assume that there is only one prosate event (if any) per each individual man and not that one man has multiple prostate events. In actuality, each prostate event probably occurs in the same men. For example, a man with acute retention is likely to have an increase in IPSS score as well. This explains why individual prostate events are not higher but prostate events as a whole are [7].

7.5   Prostate Cancer (CaP) Development

Arguably the biggest historical concern regarding TTH is the risk of CaP development or progression. This notion is based on the observations that CaP is a testosterone-dependent event, with data from eunuchs and men with congenital

5-alpha reductase deficiency demonstrating no or reduced development of prostate cancer compared to the general population [12, 13]. In relation to hypogonadal men with existing prostate cancer, data from Huggins and Hodges suggested that TTH may exacerbate progression of the disease, while castration improved symptoms [1]. These findings are further supported by numerous studies which have confirmed a role for chemical/surgical castration in the management of advanced CaP. However, current data suggests that TTH does not increase CaP risk in men with low T and without an existing diagnosis of prostate cancer. Snyder et al. [6] evaluated almost 800 men randomized to placebo versus TTH for 1 year. During the study period, only one man in the TTH group and no one in the placebo group were diagnosed with CaP. In the year after the study, only two TTH men and one placebo patient were diagnosed, suggesting low rates in both patient populations and highlighting a need for longer-term follow-up to truly evaluate the risks for prostate cancer development and progression [6].

Muller et al. [14] analyzed the placebo arm of the REDUCE trial, wherein all participants underwent a prostate biopsy regardless of PSA levels [14]. All men were 50–75 years old with a prior negative biopsy and a baseline PSA between 2.5 and 10 ng/mL. A total of 3255 men in the placebo arm had a repeat biopsy during the trial and were included in this current study. TD was defined as <288 ng/dL (10 nmol/L). Overall, 25.2% of men were diagnosed with CaP, and these rates were similar in men with TD (25.5%) compared to normal T (25.1%), $p = 0.831$ [14]. On secondary analysis, results showed that higher T levels were associated with higher CaP rates only in men with TD (OR 1.23, 95% CI 1.06–1.43; $p = 0.006$). In men with normal baseline T levels, there was no association between T levels and CaP risk ($p = 0.33$) [14]. This supports the saturation model, as once the androgen receptors are maximally stimulated, there is no additional risk of prostate cancer with further addition of T.

In the 2005 meta-analysis by Calof et al., a higher rate of prostate biopsies and prostate cancer was noted among TTH men compared to placebo; however, these were not statistically significant. Specifically, prostate biopsies during the study period occurred in 2.8 per 1000 patient-years in placebo compared to 38.7 in the TTH group. The overall odds ratio was 1.87 (95% CI 0.84–4.15) [7]. Similarly, prostate cancer diagnosis was in 8.3 per 1000 patient-years in placebo and 9.2 in TTH, OR 1.09 (95% CI 0.48–2.49) [7].

The AUA Testosterone Deficiency guidelines also addressed the risk of CaP in men on TTH. A meta-analysis of 10 randomized control trials (RCT) with 2508 men was conducted. All trials compared men with TD (defined as T < 350 ng/dL or 12.14 nmol/L) who were on TTH ($n = 1372$) versus placebo ($n = 1136$). Results demonstrated that 10 TTH patients and 9 placebo patients developed CaP, demonstrating an insignificant increased risk in CaP in men on TTH (OR 1.0, 95% CI 0.36–2.8) [8].

In addition to the lack of evidence that TTH increases the risk for prostate cancer (among men with T levels above the saturation level), there are also data that indicate that increased T levels are not associated with higher grades of prostate cancer. In a series of 431 men who had TT levels obtained pre-radical prostatectomy (RP), men with Gleason 4 predominant cancer had lower overall TT levels compared to those with Gleason 3 predominance (400 versus 450 ng/dL or 12.87 versus 15.60 nmol/L, $p = 0.001$) [15]. Similarly, TD (defined as TT < 300 ng/dL or 10.40 nmol/L) was higher in Gleason 4 predominant men compared to Gleason 3 (22.9 versus 11.4%, $p = 0.002$). The inverse was also true. When comparing men with TD ($n = 62$) to normal T ($n = 369$), Gleason 4 patterns were more common in the TD group (47% versus 28%, $p = 0.003$). On multivariable analysis (MVA), TD was a predictor of Gleason 4 predominant CaP (OR 1.87, 95% CI 1.105–3.169, $p = 0.02$) [15]. Overall results suggest that TTH is not a risk factor for CaP, and T deficiency is associated with more aggressive cancer.

A smaller study found a correlation between low FT and more aggressive CaP. Hoffman et al. evaluated 117 men with CaP. TD was defined as a TT ≤ 300 ng/dL (10.40 nmol/L) or FT ≤ 1.5 ng/dL (0.05 nmol/L) [16]. Men with low FT (but not low TT) had a greater percentage of positive biopsy cores (43% in men with low FT versus 22% in men with normal FT, $p = 0.013$). Interestingly, all men in the study with Gleason ≥8 had low FT. Of the men with low FT, 11% had Gleason ≥8 disease compared to 0% in the men with normal T, $p = 0.025$ [16].

Similar findings were seen in a larger series of 937 men post-RP. In this study, they compared Gleason scores in biopsy versus RP specimen. TD was defined as TT < 300 ng/dL (10.40 nmol/L). On RP, Gleason 4 predominance was higher in the TD group at 41.7% versus 29.1% in the normal T group, $p = 0.0029$ [17]. Men with TD were also more likely to have an upgrade in Gleason score between biopsy and RP. Nearly 20.1% of men with TD were upgraded from Gleason 3 to 4 predominance compared to 11.6% of men in the normal T group, $p = 0.002$. Interestingly, the PSA levels were the same in men with TD versus normal T (PSA 8.5 ± 5.3 ng/mL versus 8.5 ± 5.5, $p = 0.72$) [17]. This is an important point, as the conventional thinking is that more aggressive CaP is seen in men with TD as their PSA is lower and falsely reassuring, which leads to a delay in diagnosis. However, this data demonstrating similar PSA levels in men with and without TD suggests an alternative mechanism for more aggressive CaP in these men.

Data also suggests higher positive margin status in men with TD. Teloken et al. [18] noted that men with TD are more likely to have positive surgical margins after RP [18]. In their study of 64 men who underwent RP, TD was defined as TT < 270 ng/dL (9.36 nmol/L). Men with TD had higher rates of positive margins (39% versus 14.6%, $p = 0.026$). When comparing T levels of men with positive versus negative margins, they found lower T levels in the men with positive margins: 284.7 ± 145.1 ng/dL (9.87 ± 5.03 nmol/L) versus 385.7 ± 205.2 (13.37 ± 7.11 nmol/L); no p-value provided [18]. However, there was no difference between men with TD and normal T in the other pathological variables such as extracapsular extension (20.3% versus 26.6%, $p = 0.25$) or seminal vesicle involvement (3.1% versus 4.7%, $p = 0.84$). The rates of men with low (≤6) versus high (≥7) Gleason scores were also similar between men with TD and normal T ($p = 0.56$ at biopsy and 0.88 on RP specimen). Similarly, distribution of pathologic stages (pT1 and pT2 versus pT3 and pT4) was the same between men with TD and normal T ($p = 0.14$) (Table 7.1) [18].

In contrast, Kim et al. [19] noted an increased risk of extracapsular extension (ECE) and biochemical recurrence (BCR) in men with TD [19]. They evaluated 60

Table 7.1 Prostate events and recommendations

Prostate events	Synthesis of available evidence	Recommendations
PSA changes	Small PSA increases can be expected after starting TTH, especially for men with lower T levels below the saturation point	Assess PSA 2–4 weeks after starting TTH. Counsel patients to expect a PSA increase initially, especially when their T is below saturation threshold
Prostate volume changes	T levels are not correlated with prostate volume unless T is below the saturation threshold. TTH does not appear to increase prostate volume overall	Counsel patients that TTH should not impact prostate volume unless they have very low baseline T levels
LUTS	There is no evidence that TTH increase LUTS as measured by IPSS or uroflow	Reassure patients that TTH should not impact their urinary function
CaP development	Current data suggests that men receiving TTH do not have an increased risk of CaP development. Data suggests that men with TD can have more aggressive CaP	Discuss with patients that while TTH is not associated with increased risk of CaP, some evidence suggests that TD is associated with more aggressive CaP

men post-RP; 21 had TD, defined as <300 ng/dL (10.4 nmol/L) and 39 had normal T. ECE was higher in the TD group at 61.9% versus 28.2% in men with normal T ($p = 0.011$). BCR was also higher in the TD group at 23.8% compared to 5.1% in men with normal T ($p = 0.032$). On MVA of ECE, TD was a significant risk factor (OR 4.96, 95% CI 1.41–17.38, $p = 0.012$). Similarly, TD was also identified as a predictor of BCR on MVA (OR 13.64, 95% CI 1.66–2.43, $p = 0.015$) [19].

In the analysis by Muller et al. [14] of the placebo arm of the REDUCE trial, the authors did not find a link between T levels and CaP aggressiveness. The men in this study who were diagnosed with CaP were categorized into three Gleason categories: ≤6, 7, and ≥8. The median T levels in each group were similar ($p = 0.72$), suggesting that TD is not associated with higher Gleason scores [14]. On MVA of high-risk CaP, there was no association between T levels (as quintiles) and high risk CaP ($p \geq 0.1$ for all) [14]. While these findings seem to contradict the consensus in the literature, the study design may explain this. In this trial, these men were only included if they had a negative biopsy at baseline. They then underwent repeat biopsies at years 2 and 4 of the study regardless of PSA levels [14]. In contrast, most of the other studies specifically look at men diagnosed with CaP and then evaluate their T levels.

7.6   Conclusion

In summary, the role of T and prostate events, such as increased PSA, prostate volume, LUTS, or CaP, is variably defined, with relatively limited, short-term studies with small patient numbers available. Overall, there is a minor association with PSA levels and T in most men. As explained by the saturation model, PSA and T levels are most strongly correlated at T levels below the saturation threshold. Beyond the saturation point, the correlation between T and PSA is less pronounced and remains debatable. Similarly, prostate volume does not correlate with T levels beyond the saturation point, and there are no data to suggest an association with LUTS and T levels. With regard to CaP, the literature does not support a link between TTH and CaP risk, particularly among men with baseline levels beyond the saturation point. In contrast, TD seems to be associated with higher risk of CaP and higher grade and/ or pathologic features compared to men with normal T. Thus, the currently available data suggests that TTH does not increase the risk for prostate cancer among men who do not have any evidence for existing prostate cancer.

References

1. Huggins C, Hodges CV. The effects of castration, of estrogen and of androgen injection on serum phosphatases in metastatic carcinoma of the prostate. Cancer Res. 1941;1:293–7.
2. Morgentaler A, Traish AM. Shifting the paradigm of testosterone and prostate cancer: the saturation model and the limits of androgen-dependent growth. Eur Urol. 2009;55(2):310–20.
3. Khera M, Crawford D, Morales A, Salonia A, Morgentaler A. A new era of testosterone and prostate cancer: from physiology to clinical implications. Eur Urol. 2014;65(1):115–23.
4. Khera M, Bhattacharya RK, Blick G, Kushner H, Nguyen D, Miner MM. Changes in prostate specific antigen in hypogonadal men after 12 months of testosterone replacement therapy: support for the prostate saturation theory. J Urol. 2011;186(3):1005–11.
5. Marks LS, Mazer NA, Mostaghel E, et al. Effect of testosterone replacement therapy on prostate tissue in men with late-onset hypogonadism: a randomized controlled trial. JAMA. 2006;296(19):2351–61.
6. Snyder PJ, Bhasin S, Cunningham GR, et al. Effects of testosterone treatment in older men. N Engl J Med. 2016;374(7):611–24.
7. Calof OM, Singh AB, Lee ML, et al. Adverse events associated with testosterone replacement in middle-aged and older men: a meta-analysis of randomized, placebo-controlled trials. J Gerontol A Biol Sci Med Sci. 2005;60(11):1451–7.
8. Mulhall JP, Trost LW, Brannigan RE, et al. Evaluation and management of testosterone deficiency: AUA guideline. J Urol. 2018;200(2):423–32.
9. Liu CC, Huang SP, Li WM, et al. Relationship between serum testosterone and measures of benign prostatic hyperplasia in aging men. Urology. 2007;70(4):677–80.
10. Behre HM, Bohmeyer J, Nieschlag E. Prostate volume in testosterone-treated and untreated hypogonadal men in comparison to age-matched normal controls. Clin Endocrinol (Oxf). 1994;40(3):341–9.
11. Barry MJ, Fowler FJ Jr, O'Leary MP, et al. The American Urological Association symptom index for benign prostatic hyperplasia. The measurement Committee of the American Urological Association. J Urol. 1992;148(5):1549–57; discussion 1564.
12. Stocking JJ, Fiandalo MV, Pop EA, Wilton JH, Azabdaftari G, Mohler JL. Characterization of prostate cancer in a functional eunuch. J Natl Compr Canc Netw. 2016;14(9):1054–60.
13. Imperato-McGinley J, Gautier T, Zirinsky K, et al. Prostate visualization studies in males homozygous and heterozygous for 5 alpha-reductase deficiency. J Clin Endocrinol Metab. 1992;75(4):1022–6.

14. Muller RL, Gerber L, Moreira DM, Andriole G, Castro-Santamaria R, Freedland SJ. Serum testosterone and dihydrotestosterone and prostate cancer risk in the placebo arm of the Reduction by Dutasteride of Prostate Cancer Events trial. Eur Urol. 2012;62(5):757–64.
15. Botto H, Neuzillet Y, Lebret T, Camparo P, Molinie V, Raynaud JP. High incidence of predominant Gleason pattern 4 localized prostate cancer is associated with low serum testosterone. J Urol. 2011;186(4):1400–5.
16. Hoffman MA, DeWolf WC, Morgentaler A. Is low serum free testosterone a marker for high grade prostate cancer? J Urol. 2000;163(3):824–7.
17. Pichon A, Neuzillet Y, Botto H, et al. Preoperative low serum testosterone is associated with high-grade prostate cancer and an increased Gleason score upgrading. Prostate Cancer Prostatic Dis. 2015;18(4):382–7.
18. Teloken C, Da Ros CT, Caraver F, Weber FA, Cavalheiro AP, Graziottin TM. Low serum testosterone levels are associated with positive surgical margins in radical retropubic prostatectomy: hypogonadism represents bad prognosis in prostate cancer. J Urol. 2005;174(6):2178–80.
19. Kim HJ, Kim BH, Park CH, Kim CI. Usefulness of preoperative serum testosterone as a predictor of extraprostatic extension and biochemical recurrence. Korean J Urol. 2012;53(1):9–13.

Chapter 8
Testosterone in Females

Sarah Cipriani, Elisa Maseroli, and Linda Vignozzi

8.1 Introduction

Despite the fact that testosterone (T) has always been considered as the "king" of male sexuality, androgens are the most abundant steroids found also in women throughout their lifespan, playing an important role in maintaining bone metabolism, cognition, and sexual function. This chapter reviews androgens' production and fields of action in pre- and postmenopausal women, the characteristics and possible consequences of androgen deficiency, and finally the effects, management, and safety of androgen therapy in women.

8.2 Physiology of Androgens in Women

8.2.1 Production and Signaling

Androgens are 19-carbon steroids synthesized from cholesterol. The four major androgens that circulate in women during their reproductive age are listed in descending order of serum concentrations: dehydroepiandrosterone (DHEA, which principally circulates as a sulfate, DHEAS), androstenedione, T, and 5α-dihydrotestosterone (5α-DHT) [1]. Additionally, androstenediol is produced to a lesser extent [2]. DHEA and androstenedione can be considered as prohormones, which are synthesized in the ovaries and in the adrenal glands, and require conversion to T or 5α-DHT to exert their androgenic effects [3, 4]. In the ovaries, adrenal

S. Cipriani · E. Maseroli · L. Vignozzi (✉)
Andrology, Women's Endocrinology and Gender Incongruence Unit, Department of Experimental, Clinical, and Biomedical Sciences "Mario Serio", University of Florence, Florence, Italy
e-mail: linda.vignozzi@unifi.it

© Springer Nature Switzerland AG 2021
J. P. Mulhall et al. (eds.), *Controversies in Testosterone Deficiency*,
https://doi.org/10.1007/978-3-030-77111-9_8

glands, and peripheral tissues, DHEA and androstenedione are converted to T, which in turn can be transformed into 5α-DHT, the most potent androgen characterized by a three- to fivefold higher binding affinity for the androgen receptor (AR) than T [5] (Fig. 8.1). T mostly circulates protein-bound, mainly to sex hormone binding globulin (SHBG); it follows that any factor influencing the concentration of this protein (e.g., oral contraceptives) is able to affect the free/active T ratio. On the other hand, 5α-DHT is mainly an intracellular androgen, produced by the 5α-reduction of T within target cells, where it exerts its biological functions. Therefore, its serum concentration is relatively low. Additionally, androgens represent the obligatory precursors of natural estrogens that are produced mainly in ovaries and peripheral tissues and at lower levels in adrenal glands [6]. The characteristics of androgen production in women are summarized in Table 8.1.

The mechanism of action of androgens consists of the binding of T or 5α-DHT to the intracellular AR in target tissues, thus inducing conformational changes in the receptor, which separates from the heat shock proteins (HSPs), dimerizes, and translocates into the nucleus. Once bound to specific DNA regions – the androgen responsive elements (AREs) – the hormone-receptor complex elicits the activation of transcription factors, coactivators, and corepressors that modulate RNA expression of specific androgen-responsive genes, and consequently protein synthesis and cellular metabolism [2].

The main androgen secreted by the adrenal glands is DHEA, synthesized from cholesterol by the subsequent action of CYP11 and CYP17 enzymes. Testosterone is synthesized from cholesterol in the ovaries and adrenal glands and from circulating DHEA in peripheral tissues. Testosterone and androstenedione are the necessary

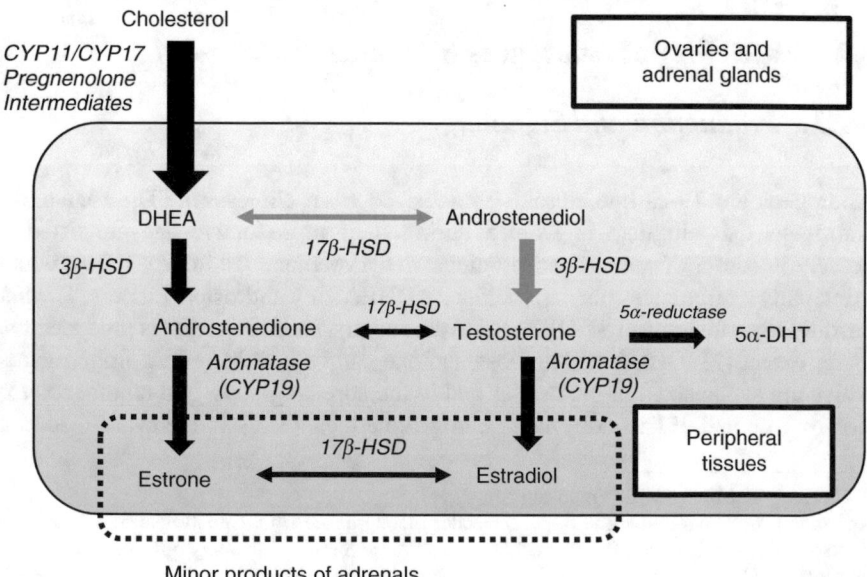

Fig. 8.1 Synthesis of androgens. (Adapted from [2])

Table 8.1 Characteristics of androgen production in women [4]

Androgen	Daily production rate	Circulating levels	Origin of production
DHEAS	3.5–20 mg	75–375 mcg/dL (2–10 micromol/L)	100% adrenal gland
DHEA	6–8 mg	0.2–0.9 mcg/dL (7–31 nmol/L)	50% adrenal gland 20% ovary 30% peripheral conversion of DHEAS
Androstenedione	1.4–6.2 mg	160–200 ng/dL (5.6–7 nmol/L)	50% adrenal gland 50% ovary
Testosterone	0.1–0.4 mg	20–60 ng/dL (0.7–2.08 nmol/L)	25% adrenal gland 25% ovary 50% peripheral conversion of androstenedione
DHT	Variable	0.1 nmol/L	100% peripheral conversion of testosterone

precursors to the synthesis of estradiol and estrone. Estrogens are a minor product of the adrenal glands (dashed rectangle). Androstenedione also can be transformed by aromatase into estrone, and interconversion between estradiol and estrone is mediated by different isoforms of 17β-HSD (17β-HSD1 and 17β-HSD2). 5α-DHT is synthesized in target tissues from testosterone by the action of 5α-reductases. Major pathways of synthesis in humans are denoted by black arrows and minor pathways are represented by gray arrows.

CYP = cytochrome P450; DHEA = dehydroepiandrosterone; DHT = dihydrotestosterone; HSD = hydroxysteroid dehydrogenase.

8.2.2   Androgens' Levels in Menopause and Aging

Androgens' production, and that of sex steroids in general, is not constant during different phases of women's life. Low levels of T primarily affect sexual differentiation of the genitalia and of the brain during fetal life. Also, it participates in the development of some secondary sexual characteristics during puberty and sexual maturation, contributing to their functional maintenance in adulthood [7]. Androgens reach their highest serum concentration in women of ages 20–30 years; then, their level gradually declines as a function of age [8]. The majority of evidence suggests that, throughout physiological menopause, estrogens synthesis rapidly decreases. However, this process is not accompanied by a concurrent drastic decrease in serum androgen levels, although it is well known that postmenopausal age is characterized by significantly lower levels of these hormones [9]. Ovarian T production remains relatively stable after natural menopause, thus increasing the percentage of overall T production derived from the ovary [10]. This phenomenon is attributable to the

menopausal-related increase in the levels of gonadotropins that stimulate steroidogenesis in ovarian hilar and stromal cells [11]. As a matter of fact, postmenopausal
women who underwent oophorectomy show a 40–50% decrease in serum T concentration [12]. Moreover, a recent cross-sectional study (measuring sex steroids by
liquid chromatography-tandem mass spectrometry, LC-MS) showed that in women
older than 70 years, serum DHEA levels are actually lower than in premenopausal
women, while total T concentrations are comparable to those seen in premenopausal
women and they even slightly increase beyond age 70 years [13].

8.3   The Role of Androgens in Women

In addition to being the necessary precursors for the biosynthesis of estrogens,
androgens exert AR-mediated effects also in women. However, while their role in
male reproductive development and function is well established, their actions in
several aspects of women's physiology remain to be fully elucidated.

Follicular Development   In ovaries, androgens are produced by the thecal cells in
response to luteinizing hormone (LH). Besides being the substrate for estrogens
synthesis, they seem to play a direct role in follicular development and consequently
in women fertility. Specifically, a proper androgen balance contributes to promote
follicle growth and prevent follicular atresia. Indeed, excess of androgens (e.g., in
polycystic ovary syndrome, PCOS) leads to a failed production of multiple follicles,
while their insufficiency has been associated with inadequate follicular development [14]. Consistent with this observation, androgen supplementation has been
exploited with the aim of increasing follicular recruitment in assisted reproductive
technology (ART), and in a recent meta-analysis, DHEA or transdermal T emerged
as a relevant adjuvant treatment. DHEA induced the best clinical pregnancy rate,
and transdermal T was associated with the highest number of embryos trans-
ferred [15].

Sexual Behavior – *Central Mechanisms*   In women, sexuality is the result of a
complex interaction of psychic, relational, social, and organic factors. Among
organic factors, sex steroids play the role of neuromodulators in brain regions that
are important for the control and for the initiation of sexual activity. While estradiol
and progesterone have been recognized for a long time as fundamental factors for a
full expression of behavioral responses related to appetitive and consummatory
phases in the female sexual response of some preclinical models, the pivotal role of
androgens as regulators of female sexual behavior has been brought into focus only
recently. Both preclinical and clinical studies demonstrate the facilitator role of
androgens in every phase of sexual response, particularly stimulating sexual desire
and neuronal pathways linked to the "reward system" [16]. Most of preclinical evidence regarding the effects of androgens on female sexual behavior derive from
studies conducted on ovariectomized female rats, which are considered the best

reference animal models to investigate hormonal and pharmacological modulations of female sexual response. In particular, in such a model, it has been demonstrated that T alone [17], as well as T combined with an aromatase inhibitor [18] and the non-aromatizable DHT [19] are able to exert an enhancing effect on both appetitive and consummatory phases of the sexual response. These observations strongly suggest that aromatization of T into estradiol is not an essential step in regulating sexual drive by T. Consistently with this line of preclinical evidence, there are three large population studies demonstrating consistent relations between androgens levels and sexual interest and arousal in women. The first one reports an association between low sexual desire, sexual arousal, or sexual responsiveness with a DHEAS value below the 10th centile for age [20]; in the second one, the frequency of sexual desire was positively associated with T [21]; in the third one, sexual desire was positively associated with T, DHEA, and androstenedione [22].

Nonreproductive Functions Since ARs in women are located in other tissues different from genital organs as well, including brain, breast, skin, adipose tissue, muscle, vasculature, and bone, androgens seem to play also nonreproductive functions [4]. In more detail, a role of androgens in the regulation of body composition as well as mood and cognition has been suggested, but corresponding evidence is still controversial, requiring further investigation [23].

8.4 Neurobiology of Testosterone

As previously mentioned, the neurofunctional modulation of the central "reward system" appears as the principal mechanism through which androgens contribute to maintain optimal levels of sexual desire, to stimulate sexual motivation, and to influence sexual gratification. The reward circuit is represented by a complex network of neural pathways involved in the process of conditioning, motivation, and emotional responses and memory, which are fundamental for both sexual and reproductive behaviors [24]. Amygdala, orbitofrontal cortex, and ventral striatum are the main cerebral areas acting in this pathway. In a recent double-blind RCT comparing healthy women treated with a gonadotropin releasing hormone (GnRH) agonist (determining a decrease in sex steroids) with those receiving placebo, the study of magnetic resonance imaging during a gambling task revealed an attenuate amygdala responsivity to pecuniary reward, reflecting a reduced involvement in positive experiences in the GnRH agonist arm [25]. Moreover, cerebral reactivity has been demonstrated to be positively associated with individual variations in T serum concentrations but not in that of estradiol. Besides, evidence suggests that androgen administration is able to modulate the neural reward pathway in studies assessing the mechanisms of anabolic steroids addiction [26]. More in detail, preclinical data show that androgens act on the reward system via dopaminergic pathways; indeed, the "conditioned spatial preference" inducted by T was blocked when a D1 or D2 dopaminergic antagonist was injected into the nucleus accumbens of adult male rats

[27]. Noteworthy, a newly identified rapid T signaling receptor (transient receptor potential melastatin 8, TRPM8) has been claimed to regulate sexual behavior while activating neurodopaminergic neurons in a mice experimental model [28].

8.5 Testosterone and Vaginal Health

ARs and enzymes involved in androgen biosynthesis were detected in different female genitourinary structures, such as vagina, clitoris, labia, bladder, urethra, vestibular glands, and pelvic floor musculature [2]. Specifically, in the vagina, they were both identified in the mucosa, submucosa, smooth muscle, stroma, and vascular endothelium. This finding suggests that androgens might play an independent role in female genitourinary physiology, along with that well-established of estrogens. As a matter of fact, local estrogens are traditionally used to treat postmenopausal vulvo-vaginal atrophy (VVA), since they have been demonstrated to stimulate proliferation and thickening of the vaginal epithelium. However, the peripheral female sexual response, consisting of sexual arousal, implies genital vasocongestion and vaginal lubrication, these processes being regulated by both androgens and estrogens [29]. Consistently, based on preclinical studies, regulation of vaginal perfusion provided by sex steroids is to be considered. Actually, estradiol and T differently influence the expression of nitric oxide (NO)-synthase and arginase, which are fundamental proteins underlying vaginal blood flow regulation, in rabbit vagina [30] and rat clitoris, where T improves the relaxation of vascular smooth muscle cells through the NO-cGMP pathway [31]. Furthermore, androgens stimulate mucification of the vaginal epithelium, which contributes to vaginal lubrication together with the estrogen-dependent production of vaginal vascular transudate [32, 33]. Noteworthy, very recently a relevant anti-inflammatory effect of the most potent AR-agonist DHT has been demonstrated in human vagina smooth muscle cells (hvSMCs) [34], opening new clinical perspectives in the management of female sexual dysfunctions (FSDs). As a matter of fact, it has been demonstrated that, in hvSMCs, DHT pre-treatment inhibited lipopolysaccharide (LPS)-induced mRNA expression of several pro-inflammatory mediators (i.e., cyclooxygenase-2, COX2; interleukin-6, IL-6; interleukin 12A, IL-12A, and interferon gamma, IFNγ), this effect being significantly blunted by AR antagonist bicalutamide and also resulting in the suppression of the IFNγ-induced immune and chronic inflammatory responses [34]. This is of particular interest, since all the steroidogenic enzymes related to androgen synthesis have been documented in rat vagina [35], paving the way for the concept of intracrinology also in the human one [36]. Actually, it has been recently published that in hvSMCs, as well as in vaginal tissue, the mRNA expression of pro-androgenic steroidogenic enzymes (13β-hydroxysteroid dehydrogenase type 1 and type 2, HSD3β1/β2; 17β-hydroxysteroid dehydrogenase type 3 and type 5, HSD17β3/β5), along with 5α-reductase isoforms and sulfo-transferase, was more abundant when compared to ovaries [36]. Moreover, in hvSMCs, the AR mRNA expression was higher than that of progestin and both estrogen receptors [36]. More pioneering, in hvSMCs, short-term DHEA supplementation increased Δ4-androstenedione levels in spent medium, as well as T and DHT secretion after longer incubation, as revealed by LC- MS analysis [36]. This study strongly demonstrates that human vagina is an androgen-target organ with the ability to synthesize androgens, thus providing new perspectives for the use of androgens against local symptoms of genito-urinary syndrome in menopause.

8.6   Testosterone and Cardiometabolic Health

The association between T and cardiometabolic health in women is still controversial, both considering endogenous T and treatment with exogenous T. The general belief is that androgens exert a pro-atherogenic effect, thus increasing the risk of cardiovascular diseases (CVD). This concept is principally based on the greater incidence of CVDs presented by men and by women with hyperandrogenism, such as those affected by PCOS. In particular, the negative impact of androgens on cardiovascular (CV) health would be explained also by a worsening in the metabolic profile, especially the lipidic and the lipoproteic ones. As a matter of fact, women with PCOS showed lower levels of high-density lipoprotein (HDL)-cholesterol and higher levels of low-density lipoprotein (LDL)-cholesterol, triglycerides, and small, dense LDL particles (sdLDL), when compared with women without PCOS, matched for body mass index (BMI) and insulin resistance [37, 38]. Noteworthy, a recent study involving 2834 postmenopausal women participating in the Multi-Ethnic Study of Atherosclerosis (MESA), higher levels of T were found to be associated with a mild increase in the CVD and coronary heart disease (CHD) risk [39].

However, hypoandrogenism seems to be detrimental for CV health as well. Indeed, there is evidence of a negative association between total T and the incidence of atherosclerosis in postmenopausal women, suggesting a contribution of reduced levels of T to the increased CV risk observed in this population [40]. On the other hand, there are studies reporting a positive association between T levels and CV events, inflammatory markers, and cardiometabolic parameters, such as C-reactive protein (CRP), blood pressure, BMI, and the presence of metabolic syndrome, thus revealing a potential pro-atherogenic effect exerted by higher endogenous T levels [41, 42].

Such evidence suggests that an optimal range of circulating T levels might affect positively CV health in women. According to this perspective, the Rancho Bernardo Study reported an U-shaped correlation between bioavailable T (bioT) and risk of coronary events in postmenopausal women, which was higher in the lowest and in the highest bioT quintiles, even after age-adjustment [43].

Additionally, some evidence suggests that physiologic T concentrations might improve endothelial function, peripheral vascular resistance, and vasomotor tone, directly acting on the vessel walls [44].

8.7 Controversies in Testosterone Deficiency in Women – Causes and Diagnosis

First of all, can we actually talk about androgen deficiency syndrome in women? Androgen deficiency is a syndrome characterized by either reduced androgen production or reduced activity and can arise in women at any age. It was considered as a well-defined clinical entity for the first time in 2002, based on the consensus reached during a meeting at the University of Princeton. According to this, female androgen deficiency is a syndrome delineated by reduced sexual desire, chronic tiredness, clinically unjustified loss of bone mass, reduction in muscle strength, reduced feeling of wellness or mood changes, thinning of hair, and altered cognition and memory [45]. However, nowadays the diagnosis of androgen deficiency poses considerable controversies, principally due to the lack of both a well-defined clinical syndrome with specific signs and symptoms and of age-based standardized reference ranges for serum T and free T concentrations.

8.7.1 Causes

There are many medical conditions identified as causes of androgen deficiency, and they are summarized in Table 8.2, together with their underlying mechanisms.

- Bilateral oophorectomy. As mentioned above, most studies show that oophorectomized women have lower total and free T levels than naturally menopausal women, since postmenopausal ovary still produces some T. Nevertheless, the literature provides contradictory evidence about this issue, leading to a conclusion that oophorectomized women definitely lack the ovarian production of T, although an androgen profile will not steadily differentiate surgical from natural menopausal women.
- Primary adrenal insufficiency. Some pathological processes affecting adrenal function may result in hypoandrogenemia, particularly consisting of reduced levels of DHEA and DHEAS, as the major source of these two androgens is the adrenal gland. However, to date, there is insufficient evidence in support of a therapeutic use of DHEA in women with adrenal insufficiency.
- Hypopituitarism. This condition can cause androgen deficiency since it can include hypogonadotropic hypogonadism and/or secondary adrenal insufficiency, thus affecting the two main sources of androgens in women. As a matter of fact, it has been demonstrated that serum T, free T, androstenedione, and DHEAS levels were markedly reduced in women with hypopituitarism (older or not than 50 years old, and receiving or not receiving treatment with estrogens) as compared to controls [46]. Moreover, androgen levels were decreased in hypopituitary women with both hypogonadism and hypoadrenalism compared with those women with hypogonadism alone [46].

Table 8.2 Causes and mechanisms of androgen insufficiency in women (adapted from [3])

Causes of androgen insufficiency	Mechanism
Spontaneous	
Physiologic decline with age from mid-to-late reproductive years	Decline in production of androgens by the ovaries and adrenal glands
Hypothalamic amenorrhea	Anovulation
Primary ovarian insufficiency/gonadal dysgenesis	Anovulation
Hyperprolactinemia	Suppression of pituitary gonadotropins; anovulation
Adrenal insufficiency	Loss of adrenal production of pre-androgens
Panhypopituitarism/hypogonadotropic hypogonadism	Loss of adrenal production of pre-androgens/ovarian production of androgens
Other medical conditions (e.g., chronic liver diseases, HIV infections, hyperthyroidism, and pregnancy)	Increased levels of SHBG reduce concentrations of free testosterone
Iatrogenic	*Mechanism*
Surgical menopause at any age	Loss of ovarian production of androgens
Chemotherapy	Ovarian failure
Radiotherapy to the pelvis	Ovarian failure
Systemic glucocorticosteroid therapy	Loss of adrenal production of pre-androgens
Drug-induced hyperprolactinemia	Suppression of pituitary gonadotropins; anovulation
Systemic hormonal contraception	Reduction of ovarian production of androgens; increased levels of SHBG reduce concentrations of free testosterone
Oral non-contraceptive therapy (e.g., phenobarbital, phenytoin, carbamazepine, and thyroxine), ethanol	Increased levels of SHBG reduce concentrations of free testosterone

- Premature ovarian insufficiency (POI). POI is defined as a premature decrease in ovarian function occurring before the age of 40, which is caused by different pathologic/iatrogenic conditions affecting the ovaries. It is typically characterized by hypergonadotropic hypogonadism, associated with estrogen deficiency. Besides, women with POI may present with androgen deficiency due to the ovarian cortex atrophy, as well. Since this last point has not been well established, Soman and colleagues recently published a systematic review and meta-analysis whose aim was to investigate serum androgen profiles of women with POI. They concluded that this population presented with significantly lower serum concentrations of total T, DHEAS, and androstenedione when compared with fertile controls (being SHBG levels comparable between the two groups), but with higher levels of DHEA when compared with natural postmenopausal women [47].
- Anorexia nervosa (AN). AN is an eating disorder complicated by endocrine abnormalities, including hypogonadotropic hypogonadism. In a study conducted on more than 200 affected women, total and free T, but not DHEAS,

concentrations were lower than in controls [48]. These results support the hypothesis that, in anorexic women, a reduction in the ovarian androgens production (due to the hypogonadotropic hypogonadism), and not that of adrenal androgen precursors, is the principal contributor to their overall androgen deficiency.

- Medications. Several medications may cause a relative androgen deficiency through different mechanisms. Glucocorticoid may determine adrenal androgen suppression [49, 50]. Drugs inducing hyperprolactinemia (e.g., phenothiazines and butyrophenones) lead to suppression of pituitary gonadotropins, thus abolishing their simulating effect on ovarian hormonal production. Systemic hormonal contraception and hormonal replacement therapy for menopause may both suppress ovarian androgen production and reduce serum free T concentrations by increasing serum SHBG levels. However, although there is biological plausibility to this concept, there is no compelling evidence that oral contraceptive-induced androgen deficiency by ovarian suppression has to be clinically significant.

- Human immunodeficiency virus (HIV) infection. Low androgen levels have been reported in HIV-positive women [51, 52], but there is conflicting evidence derived from placebo-controlled studies investigating the effectiveness of T therapy in this female population.

8.7.2 Diagnostic Controversies

The 2014 Endocrine Society (ES) guidelines on Androgen Therapy in Women recommend against making a clinical diagnosis of androgen deficiency syndrome in healthy women, because of the lack of criteria for a well-defined syndrome [23]. Moreover, in women, there is no availability of an universally accepted and age-standardized reference range of androgen serum concentrations that would allow to make a biochemical diagnosis of hypoandrogenism underlying FSD or to establish if a woman is eligible for T treatment or not. This issue is also due to the fact that the immunoassay (IA) methods, which are the most frequently used T measurement technique in clinical practice, show poor accuracy in detecting the physiological low androgen concentrations seen in women (<1,5–2 nM). In addition, it should be considered that only 1–2% of circulating total T is biologically active, because of its high affinity binding to SHBG, and that serum concentrations of this protein are extremely variable, depending on intercurrent medications or diseases, such as oral contraceptives, hyperthyroidism, or liver diseases. Finally, circulating levels of T do not necessarily reflect the real exposure of peripheral tissues to androgens. As a matter of fact, tissue sensitivity to these hormones displays an important inter-individual variability, based on genetic differences in the distribution and sensitivity of the AR and in the distribution and activity of 5α-reductase and aromatase in peripheral tissues [3].

8.7.3 Role of Testosterone Measurement Assays

T measurement plays a crucial role in the controversies related to female androgen deficiency diagnosis. Most of the current IA methods for total T have been optimized for male T measurements, but they are, at best, marginal when applied to women, even when used to diagnose hyperandrogenism [53]. Indeed, it is well known from the literature that IA methods are relatively inaccurate and they lack of the low-end sensitivity requirements for measuring the low T levels usually encountered in healthy women, even more when used for investigating female androgen deficiency syndromes. In order to overcome this issue, in recent years, researchers have turned to ultrasensitive methods employing mass spectrometry coupled to either gas chromatography or high-performance liquid chromatography. To date, LC-MS is considered to be the most sensitive approach for measuring sex steroid concentrations [54], although the development of a true inter-method standardization in different MS laboratories is needed to promote this technique to accepted routine method in both clinical and reference laboratories [55]. Furthermore, when evaluating hypoandrogenemia in women, measurement of free T levels might be considered as well. Unfortunately, this assessment is complicated by the limitations of currently available free T assays. The gold standard is represented by the equilibrium dialysis method, but it has limited applications, since it is technically difficult, time consuming, and expensive [56]. On the contrary, direct radioimmunoassay (RIA) is widely available, but its use in clinical research has been brought into question because of inconsistent results and lack of validation in populations with binding globulin anomalies, since protein effects cannot be ruled out [57]. Lastly, a calculated value for free T, using the mass action equation, may be useful, but its accuracy depends significantly on the validity of original total T and SHBG measurements and on the variability of SHBG binding conditions, related to the overall hormonal and nutrient women's status [57].

For all the above reasons, clinicians are discouraged to pose a biochemical diagnosis of hypoandrogenemia in women, especially in relative androgen deficiency states [23, 58]. However, in the last few years, more sensitive T measurement methods employing tandem MS have become more accessible, and a reference method and reference standards are now available at the Centers for Disease Control and Prevention (http://www.cdc.gov/labstandards/hs.html) [59].

8.8 Controversies in Testosterone Deficiency in Women – Therapy

Once the diagnosis of female androgen deficiency is suspected, the question becomes: is it treatable and how? – Although FSD includes a multifactorial range of concerns, research on androgen therapy for women has been mainly centered on the treatment of low desire. Therefore, based on evidence suggesting that androgens decline with aging, as well as with oophorectomy, and that endogenous concentrations of androgens are positively associated with female sexual function, natural and surgical menopausal women have represented the main target-study population of the majority of research on T treatment.

8.8.1 Systemic Testosterone Therapy for HSDD in Postmenopausal Women

According to the Diagnostic and Statistical Manual of Mental Disorders (DSM) IV and IV-TR, HSDD in women is essentially defined as the absence of sexual fantasies and desire for sexual activity, causing distress. Successively, in DSM V, it has been merged with female sexual arousal disorder, and they were labeled together as female sexual interest–arousal disorder (FSIAD), nevertheless remaining principally based on sexual desire [60]. The 2014 Clinical Practice Guideline from the ES suggests a 3- to 6-month trial of T therapy for postmenopausal women who request treatment for properly diagnosed HSDD and who do not present any contraindications to it [23]. Consistently, HSDD in postmenopausal women represents the only evidence-based indication for the use of T in females, supported by a biopsychosocial assessment and treatment model, also according to the more recent Global Consensus Position Statement on the Use of Testosterone Therapy for Women, published in 2019 [58]. As a matter of fact, studies enrolling both natural and surgical postmenopausal women using transdermal T, either alone or combined with estrogens, showed considerable efficacy in the treatment of HSDD [61–63]. This finding has been recently corroborated by a systematic review and meta-analysis reporting a better efficacy of transdermal T therapy than placebo in postmenopausal women [64]. Noteworthy, four 24-week phase 3 clinical trials conducted in physiologically and oophorectomized menopausal women with HSDD demonstrated a significant improvement in sexual desire and in the frequency of satisfying sexual events vs. placebo in those treated with a 300 mcg/day T transdermal patch (TTP) [61, 65–67]. Additionally, three of the four studies reported a significant amelioration of sexually related distress in women receiving T (65–68% decrease in distress) vs. placebo (only 40–48% decrease). Of great importance, a very recent systematic review and meta-analysis of RCT data, comprising 8480 participants, showed that, compared with placebo or a with a comparator (e.g., estrogen, with or without progestogen), T significantly increased sexual function, including satisfactory sexual event frequency, sexual desire, pleasure, arousal, orgasm, responsiveness, and self-image, and reduced sexual concerns and distress in postmenopausal women [68].

In 2006, T therapy was previously approved in Europe for the treatment of HSDD in surgical menopausal women, in form of a 300 mcg/day TTP (trade name Intrinsa®), but voluntarily withdrawn in 2012 by the manufacturer for commercial reasons [69]. The Food and Drug Administration (FDA) then withheld the approval of this T formulation based on concerns about long-term negative effects that actually had not been reported during clinical use in the European Union. Additionally, a transdermal gel (Libigel ®, BioSante) underwent FDA evaluation but it failed to show greater efficacy compared to placebo. A 1% T cream (Androfeme®, Lawley Pharmaceuticals) is currently available in Australia for symptoms associated with T deficiency, such as low sexual desire (recommended dose 0.5 g/day). As a result, in most countries, including Europe and the United States, T formulations for women are not commercially available. The only options available for clinicians are to prescribe compounded formulations provided by pharmacies (e.g., ointments and creams) or those approved for the treatment of male hypogonadism (intramuscular injections, subcutaneous implants, transdermal patches, and gels), modified to much lower administered doses (usually one-tenth of the male dosing). The use of the latter in women involves breaking of tablets and cutting of patches or using portions of gel products, with imprecision possibly leading to sub-optimal dosing or overdosing. Particularly, oral T formulations show an important variation in absorption that may result in hepatotoxicity and cardiac side effects due to androgen excess. Transdermal products appear to be the best choice for T treatment in women, providing an appropriate balance between serum T concentrations and safety profile. Nevertheless, the ES guidelines suggest against the treatment of women with either preparations formulated for men or those formulated by pharmacies, since safety and efficacy of most compounded T products are unknown and they can easily lead to supraphysiological serum T levels and, eventually, to virilization [23].

8.8.2 Other Effects of Testosterone Therapy

8.8.2.1 Mood and Well-Being

While only few studies investigated how T therapy influences mood in women as the primary outcome, and/or in samples properly diagnosed for depression, a number of RCTs showed an improvement in mood as a secondary endpoint in women not screened for depression before enrollment. In one of these RCTs – evaluating the use of transdermal T vs. placebo in postmenopausal women with HSDD – a significant improvement in psychological well-being resulted in the T arm [62]. A similar finding was obtained in an RCT – involving premenopausal women with low libido and without evidence of severe clinical depression on the Beck Depression Inventory (BDI) – randomized to T cream (10 mg/day) or placebo [70]. In particular, the T cream arm showed statistically significant improvements in the composite scores of the Psychological General Well-Being Index and the Sabbatsberg Sexual Self-Rating Scale, in addition to a mean decrease in BDI score approaching significance, compared with placebo. Only two small pilot studies have investigated T as augmentation therapy for standard treatment in resistant depression, one using methyltestosterone and the other a TTP, respectively, and both reported positive results [71, 72]. In contrast, in different meta-analyses exploring the potential benefits of T therapy on outcomes different from sexual functioning, such as cognitive function, mood, bone mineral density (BMD), and vasomotor symptoms, no evidence of beneficial effects for any of these endpoints was observed [68, 73, 74].

8.8.2.2 Cardiovascular Health

Concerning thromboembolic risk, T treatment has been associated with an increase in hematocrit, giving rise to the risk of polycythemia and thromboembolic events [75]. Moreover, it has been reported that T therapy can influence the lipid profile, strongly depending on the route of administration, dosage, and concomitant use of estrogens, with oral formulations showing the most adverse effects. This could be explained by the first pass effect on the liver characteristic of the oral administration. In fact, oral methyltestosterone administered with oral estrogens is associated with decreased HDL [76, 77] and apolipoprotein A1 levels [76] in different studies, although in other studies, it also potentially decreased atherogenic protein fractions, such as triglycerides, apolipoprotein IIIC [77], and apolipoprotein B [78]. A recent meta-analysis found a significant rise in LDL-cholesterol as well as a reduction of total cholesterol and HDL-cholesterol along with triglycerides levels with oral, but not with non-oral, T formulations [68]. There are data about T subcutaneous implants [79], transdermal patches [80], or sprays [81] not reporting adversely altered lipid profile, CRP, glycated hemoglobin (HbA1c), or insulin sensitivity. In two large studies, APHRODITE [80] and ADORE [63], evaluating natural postmenopausal women mostly taking transdermal T alone (150 or 300 mcg/day TTPs), no adverse changes in either lipid or lipoprotein levels were detected. In agreement with these observations, in a systematic review by Spoletini et al., investigating the relationship between androgens and CV diseases in postmenopausal women [82], the authors highlighted that androgen replacement therapy (methyltestosterone, T implants, transdermal T, or DHEA) did not negatively influence, and in some cases it even improved, the metabolic profile in women after menopause. Only one among the reviewed studies showed the reverse, reporting that, in postmenopausal women, T undecanoate negatively affected lipid profile and insulin sensitivity [83]. However, the long-term consequences of the possible lipid profile alterations are unknown.

When looking specifically at CVDs, there are no sufficient long-term prospective studies to definitively assess the relationship between exogenous T administration and CV risk in women [84]. Actually, none of the RCTs comparing transdermal T therapy with placebo showed a difference in event rate for any CVD outcome, as well as in venous thromboembolic events in short-term studies [23, 68]. Accordingly, a 4-year open-label extension of two clinical trials based on the use of 300 mcg/day TTP in 967 oophorectomized women, treated with a concomitant estrogen therapy, showed no increase over time in the rate of new occurrences or severity of adverse events [85]. Lastly, almost all studies agree that T does not significantly affect systolic and diastolic blood pressure as compared to placebo [58, 86, 87].

8.8.2.3 Bone and Body Composition

It has been reported that endogenous androgen levels correlate with trabecular and cortical bone mass density (BMD) in women, particularly in women aged ≥60 years [88]. The effects of low-dose androgen administration with or without estrogens on BMD have been studied mostly in small size trials, with a short duration. In a small RCT, conducted on hypopituitary women with severe androgen deficiency, transdermal T (300 mcg/day) increased BMD at the hip and radius but not at the spine [89]. In a randomized trial, enrolling surgical postmenopausal women, a combined therapy of methyltestosterone (2.5 mg/day) plus estrogens was able to increase spine and hip BMD, as compared with the estrogen-alone arm [76]. In contrast, studies enrolling natural postmenopausal women are conflicting, since some demonstrate positive effects on BMD of T combined with estrogens [90, 91], while others report no advantages [92]. Moreover, no RCT has investigated the effect of T treatment on fracture risk. However, a recent meta-analysis showed that T treatment has no effects on body composition and musculoskeletal health in women [68]. Similar results were reported for cognitive functions. In conclusion, due to the small number of women who contributed data for these outcomes, the effects of T on musculoskeletal and cognitive health definitively warrant further investigation.

8.8.3   Local Androgen Therapy

Off-label T preparations include topical therapies, such as compounded local creams. An example of commercially available formulation is a T propionate cream, 1–2% in white petroleum jelly, that should be applied daily to the clitoris and labia minora. Regarding the evidence about local T therapy efficacy, only few small studies are relevant [93–95]. In 20 women receiving vaginal 0.5 mg 2% T with 0.625 mg conjugated equine estrogens twice a week, this combined therapy was more effective than local estrogens alone in improving multiple sexuality scores, including intensity of desire [96]. In another study conducted on 10 women with breast cancer undergoing aromatase inhibitor treatment, the use of 300 mcg/day vaginal T for 4 weeks repaired vaginal cytology and blunted dyspareunia, with serum T levels remaining within the normal premenopausal range [97]. However, further studies are needed to assess the efficacy and safety of local T formulations, whose use is generally discouraged because of the lack of standardization in their kinetics of absorption and in the T concentrations ranges provided.

An intravaginal formulation of synthetic DHEA (prasterone vaginal ovules, 6.5 mg/day) was recently approved by the FDA and then by the European Medical Agency (EMA) for the treatment of moderate to severe dyspareunia related to VVA in postmenopausal women. However, although it is not properly approved for the treatment of FSD, recent evidence highlights the benefits of the local therapy with DHEA on quality of life and all domains of sexual dysfunction, including bothersome symptoms such as dyspareunia and vaginal dryness, as compared with placebo [98, 99]. Moreover, different studies reported that intravaginal administration of DHEA over a 12-week period was able to reduce vaginal pH and improve the vaginal maturity index (VMI) when compared with placebo, thus inducing an improvement in the physical appearance of the vagina in menopausal women [98, 100]. Interestingly, based on the results of the phase III ERC-231 and -238 trials for the approval of prasterone, during 52 weeks of treatment, changes in serum levels of T and estradiol increased from baseline but remained well within the limits of normal postmenopausal women [101]. Ultimately, intravaginal prasterone is an effective and generally well-tolerated option for the treatment of genitourinary syndrome of menopause (GSM), and further studies are required to compare its efficacy with vaginal estrogens and assess its local anti-inflammatory potential, in the light of the innovative insights on intracrinology got from recent preclinical studies [36].

8.8.4   Management and Safety

According to the current guidelines' recommendations [23, 58], in women who are appropriate candidates for T therapy, baseline T level should be checked and an approved non-oral formulation for women (transdermal patch, cream, or gel) should be used if such a preparation is available. If not, it is reasonable to prescribe an off-label approved male formulation or a compounded product, the latter on the condition that it is provided by a compounding pharmacy compliant with purity of Active Pharmaceutical Ingredients and Good Manufacturing Practice. In any case, provided hormone concentrations should be maintained in the physiologic premenopausal female range. There is no T concentration representing a treatment goal for replacement therapy, as T serum levels do not predict treatment efficacy. T levels should be monitored 3–6 weeks after initiation of therapy and then every 4–6 months, in order to exclude an overuse or signs of androgen excess. Cessation of therapy is suggested for women without treatment response within 6 months. Notably, safety and efficacy data for T therapy in women are only available within 24 months.

First, potential side effects of T therapy include signs of hyperandrogenism, i.e., acne, hirsutism, androgenic alopecia, and deepening of the voice. However, they are dose dependent and uncommon if physiological hormone levels are maintained. In placebo-controlled studies, women receiving transdermal T treatment up to 12 months reported a higher frequency of masculinizing effects, mainly increased body hair growth [66, 80, 102]. In the APHRODITE study, only the 300 mcg/day T dose was associated with a higher rate of hair growth [80]. Clitoromegaly has not been highlighted as an adverse effect of transdermal therapy across different studies.

Second, the risk of hormone-dependent tumors has to be taken into account. To date, the relation between androgens and risk of breast cancer remains unclear. Preclinical studies have shown that T is protective for some subtypes of breast cancer [103], while epidemiological studies reporting positive associations between endogenous concentrations of T and risk of breast cancer present important limitations [104, 105]. In general, a number of cohort studies involving a variety of worldwide populations show a small but significant association between androgens (T, androstenedione, DHEA, and DHEAS) and postmenopausal breast cancer [106–108], but the magnitude of risk is similar to that found for estradiol and it seems to be confined to ER+/PR+ breast cancers. However, all these studies present substantial limitations. First is the assumption that T can be included in analyses as independent variable without taking into account the concentrations of estrogens and the variable amount of T aromatized to estrogens; additionally, the measurement of a single hormone is a poor proxy for lifetime exposure to it, which is characterized by age-related, cyclic, and circadian fluctuations. In the APHRODITE study, when considering a subset of women evaluated for breast density, no differences in mammographic density were seen between placebo and either 150 mcg/day or 300 mcg/day T arms [109]. Nevertheless, over a 52-week follow-up, breast cancer was diagnosed in four women receiving T (with no cases in the placebo group): in two of the four cases, the tumor likely was present before randomization, whereas the third women had a long-term history of prior estrogen use. Analyses of data from the Nurses' Health Study suggested that natural menopausal women currently taking estrogen plus methyltestosterone (a non-aromatizable synthetic androgen), but not those who had taken the combined therapy in the past, had a greater risk of breast cancer (relative risk, RR = 2.48; 95% CI, 1.53–4.0) than women using estrogens with or without progestin (RR = 1.23; 95% CI, 1.05–1.44), as compared with women who had never used hormones [110]. In contrast, a large case-control trial of women aged 50–64 years reported no alteration of breast cancer risk with methyltestosterone [111]. Two observational studies – evaluating the risk of breast cancer associated with T implant therapy and transdermal T and including similar number of patients and duration of follow-up as the Nurses' Health Study – reported that the risk for current users was comparable to the background risk in the general population [112, 113]. Similarly, a recent 10-year prospective cohort study showed that long-term therapy with T subcutaneous implants did not increase the incidence of invasive breast cancer [114]. Furthermore, across the clinical trial program for the TTP, including studies up to 2 years in duration, no increased risk of invasive breast cancer was observed [115]. In summary, available clinical trials are characterized by inappropriate size and duration to ascertain whether the observed associations between T treatment and breast cancer are causal. Consequently, clinicians choosing to prescribe T therapy should be well aware of this potential risk and should provide informed consent to patients about it.

Finally, data for the assessment of an association between exogenous T and the risk of ovarian and endometrial cancer are overall scarce. For this outcome, more data regarding endometrial effects of T therapy are available, also because the AR has been identified in the stromal compartment of postmenopausal endometrium and in the glandular compartment of endometrial cancers [116]. In a retrospective analysis on 258 postmenopausal taking both estrogens and T via subcutaneous implants, endometrial monitoring revealed that almost 66% of the sample had an endometrial polyp at hysteroscopy and 20.4% a simple hyperplasia after 2 years of treatment [117]. Concerning endometrial hyperplasia, both the effect of

T-to-estradiol conversion in altered endometrium and that of high estradiol concentrations provided by the pellets should be considered. In the APRHODITE study, no differences in endometrial events evaluated through ultrasound and endometrial biopsy were found among groups [80], although women in the 300 mcg/day T group showed a higher rate of endometrial bleeding, as compared with the 150 mcg/day and the placebo groups (10.6%, 2.7%, and 2.6%, respectively) [80]. Notably, more women on the higher T dose had an endometrial biopsy indicative of "insufficient tissue for diagnosis," thus suggesting endometrial atrophy promoted by T, which is actually believed to be associated with such an alteration when given without concomitant estrogens.

8.8.5   Recommendations for Premenopausal Women

As for postmenopausal women, women in their reproductive years often complain about decreased sexual desire, arousal, and satisfaction, which may result even more distressing given the young age, and are likely to impair intimate relationships and fertility [20, 118]. Nevertheless, premenopausal women have even fewer treatment options for FSD. Actually, there are only limited clinical trials examining the efficacy and safety of androgen therapy in this population [70, 81]. Therefore, current guidelines unanimously recommend T therapy for postmenopausal women properly diagnosed with HSDD [23, 58], while T therapy has only been listed as a potential treatment for HSDD for women in the late reproductive years by the International Society for the Study of Women's Sexual Health (ISSWSH) HSDD process of care (POC) [119].

If clinicians choose to prescribe an off-label T formulation for the treatment of distressing low sexual desire in menstruating patients, a medically acceptable form of contraception and an informed consent should be provided, since T excess might lead to virilization of a female fetus in case of pregnancy. At present, flibanserin is the only FDA-approved medication for generalized acquired HSDD in premenopausal women. This is a non-hormonal, centrally acting, multifunctional serotonin agonist and antagonist, given orally at a daily dosage of 100 mg at bedtime [120]. Flibanserin demonstrated a statistically and clinically significant improvement in sexual desire and in the number of sexually satisfying events, as well as a decrease in sexual distress as compared with placebo, in three pivotal trials including more than 3500 women [121–123], thus representing a viable alternative to T therapy.

8.8.6   Other Androgenic Preparations

Systemic DHEA Oral DHEA (25–50 mg/day) is available in the United States as a dietary supplement, and, as such, it receives only minimal regulatory oversight by the FDA. Consequently, DHEA products are considerably variable in quality and dose, although it has been demonstrated that a daily dose of 50 mg DHEA is associated with notable androgenic side effects, such as acne and hirsutism [124]. DHEA therapy has been proposed as a replacement therapy in women with primary adrenal insufficiency, when they present with significantly impaired mood or well-being despite appropriate glucocorticoid and mineralocorticoid replacement. However, clinical data on its efficacy are conflicting. Moreover, the ES guidelines suggest against the routine use of DHEA for the treatment of sexual symptoms in postmenopausal women, based upon available data. On one hand, two recent meta-analyses showed limited efficacy of DHEA in improving sexual function, quality of life, and menopausal symptoms in postmenopausal women vs. placebo, and, on the other hand, a similar effect on glycolipid profile, BMD, body weight and BMI, and an increase in androgenic side effects [73, 125].

Androstenedione As a prohormone, androstenedione is rapidly converted into T and estrone, thus increasing their serum levels, when administered orally to women [126]. However, its androgenic side effects and its impact on sexual function have not been adequately investigated yet.

8.9 Conclusions

Although a proper diagnosis of female androgen deficiency is currently controversial, there are many identifiable causes leading to a clinical condition characterized by a lack of androgen action in women. Of particular relevance is its manifestation as reduced sexual motivation and desire, which is related to aging-related androgen decline in natural menopause and abrupt cessation of androgen production in surgical menopause. A recent Global Position Statement recommends the use of T therapy in natural or surgical postmenopausal women diagnosed with HSDD (with or without concurrent estrogen therapy), when all biopsychosocial modifiable factors have been addressed [58]. Despite the need of adequately powered RCTs to further assess long-term safety of T treatment and of its pleiotropic effects, available evidence suggests a new role of T as the "queen" hormone in women sexual well-being.

References

1. Burger HG. Androgen production in women. Fertil Steril. 2002;77 Suppl 4:S3.
2. Traish AM, Vignozzi L, Simon JA, et al. Role of androgens in female genitourinary tissue structure and function: implications in the genitourinary syndrome of menopause. Sex Med Rev. 2018;6(4):558–71.
3. Davis SR, Wahlin-Jacobsen S. Testosterone in women – the clinical significance. Lancet Diabetes Endocrinol. 2015;3(12):980–92.
4. Udoff L. Overview of androgen deficiency and therapy in women. In: Marin KA, editor, UpToDate; 2019.

5. Labrie F, Martel C, Bélanger A, et al. Androgens in women are essentially made from DHEA in each peripheral tissue according to intracrinology. J Steroid Biochem Mol Biol. 2017;168:9–18.
6. Simpson ER. Aromatization of androgens in women: current concepts and findings. Fertil Steril. 2002;77 Suppl 4:S6–S10.
7. Hodgson T, Braunstein GD. Physiological effects of androgens in women. In: Azziz R, Nestler JE, Dewailly D, editors. Contemporary endocrinology: androgen excess disorders in women: polycystic ovary syndrome and other disorders. 2nd ed. Totowa: Humana Press Inc; 2007. p. 49–61.
8. Davison SL, Bell R, Donath S, et al. Androgen levels in adult females: changes with age, menopause, and oophorectomy. J Clin Endocrinol Metab. 2005;90:3847.
9. Burger HG, Dudley EC, Cui J, et al. A prospective longitudinal study of serum testosterone, dehydroepiandrosterone sulfate, and sex hormone-binding globulin levels through the menopause transition. J Clin Endocrinol Metab. 2000;85:2832–8.
10. Adashi EY. The climacteric ovary as a functional gonadotropin-driven androgen-producing gland. Fertil Steril. 1994;62:20.
11. Judd HL, Fournet N. Changes of ovarian hormonal function with aging. Exp Gerontol. 1994;29:285.
12. Laughlin GA, Barrett-Connor E, Kritz-Silverstein D, von Mühlen D. Hysterectomy, oophorectomy, and endogenous sex hormone levels in older women: the Rancho Bernardo Study. J Clin Endocrinol Metab. 2000;85:645.
13. Davis SR, Bell RJ, Robinson PJ, et al. Testosterone and estrone increase from the age of 70 years: findings from the sex hormones in older women study. J Clin Endocrinol Metab. 2019;104(12):6291–300.
14. Vendola KA, Zhou J, Adesanya OO, Weil SJ, Bondy CA. Androgens stimulate early stages of follicular growth in the primate ovary. J Clin Invest. 1998;101:2622–9.
15. Zhang Y, Zhang C, Shu J, Guo J, Chang HM, Leung PCK, Sheng JZ, Huang H. Adjuvant treatment strategies in ovarian stimulation for poor responders undergoing IVF: a systematic review and network meta-analysis. Hum Reprod Update. 2020;26(2):247–63.
16. Clayton AH, Vignozzi L. Pathophysiology and medical management of hypoactive sexual desire disorder. In: Goldstein I, Clayton AH, Goldstein AT, Kim NN, Kingsber SA, editors. Textbook of female sexual function and dysfunction - diagnosis and treatment. Oxford: Wiley Blackwell; 2018. p. 59–100.
17. Jones SL, Ismail N, Pfaus JG. Facilitation of sexual behavior in ovariectomized rats by estradiol and testosterone: a preclinical model of androgen effects on female sexual desire. Psychoneuroendocrinology. 2017;79:122–33.
18. Pfaus JG, Jones SL, Flanagan-Cato LM, et al. Female sexual behavior. In: Plant TM, Zeleznik AJ, editors. Knobil and Neill's physiology of reproduction, vol. 2. New York: Elsevier; 2015. p. 2287–370.
19. Maseroli E, Pfaus JG, Santangelo A, et al. Study on the effect of non-aromatizable androgen dihydrotestosterone (DHT) on the sexual behavior of ovariectomized female rats primed with estradiol. J Sex Med. 2019;16(6):S16–7.
20. Davis SR, Davison SL, Donath S, Bell RJ. Circulating androgen levels and self-reported sexual function in women. JAMA. 2005;294(1):91–6.
21. Wåhlin-Jacobsen S, Pedersen AT, Kristensen E, Laessøe NC, Lundqvist M, Cohen AS, Hougaard DM, Giraldi A. Is there a correlation between androgens and sexual desire in women? J Sex Med. 2015;12(2):358–73.
22. Randolph JF Jr, Zheng H, Avis NE, Greendale GA, Harlow SD. Masturbation frequency and sexual function domains are associated with serum reproductive hormone levels across the menopausal transition. J Clin Endocrinol Metab. 2015;100(1):258–66.
23. Wierman ME, Arlt W, Basson R, et al. Androgen therapy in women: a reappraisal: an endocrine society clinical practice guideline. J Clin Endocrinol Metab. 2014;99(10):3489–510.

24. Hamann S. Sex differences in the responses of the human amygdala. Neuroscientist. 2005;11(4):288–93.
25. Macoveanu J, Henningsson S, Pinborg A, et al. Sex-steroid hormone manipulation reduces brain response to reward. Neuropsychopharmacology. 2016;41(4):1057–65.
26. Mhillaj E, Morgense MG, Tucci P, et al. Effects of anabolic-androgens on brain reward function. Front Neurosci-Switz. 2015;9(295):1–13.
27. Schroeder JP, Packard MG. Role of dopamine receptor subtypes in the acquisition of a testosterone conditioned place preference in rats. Neurosci Lett. 2000;282(1–2):17–20.
28. Mohandass A, Krishnan V, Gribkova ED, et al. TRPM8 as the rapid testosterone signaling receptor: implications in the regulation of dimorphic sexual and social behaviors. FASEB J. 2020. https://doi.org/10.1096/fj.202000794R. Online ahead of print.
29. Davis S, Worsley R, Miller KK, Parish SJ, Santoro N. Androgens and female sexual function and dysfunction—findings from the Fourth International Consultation of Sexual Medicine. J Sex Med. 2016;13(2):168–78.
30. Traish AM, Kim NN, Huang YH, et al. Sex steroid hormones differentially regulate nitric oxide synthase and arginase activities in the proximal and distal rabbit vagina. Int J Impot Res. 2003;15:397–404.
31. Comeglio P, Cellai I, Filippi S, et al. Differential effects of testosterone and estradiol on clitoral function: an experimental study in rats. J Sex Med. 2016;13(12):1858–71.
32. Labrie F, Martel C, Pelletier G. Is vulvovaginal atrophy due to a lack of both estrogens and androgens? Menopause. 2017;24(4):452–61.
33. Traish AM, Botchevar E, Kim NN. Biochemical factors modulating female genital sexual arousal physiology. J Sex Med. 2010;7(9):2925–46.
34. Maseroli E, Cellai I, Filippi S, et al. Anti-inflammatory effects of androgens in the human vagina. J Mol Endocrinol. 2020;65(3):109–24.
35. Labrie F, Bélanger A, Simard J, et al. DHEA and peripheral androgen and estrogen formation: intracrinology. Ann N Y Acad Sci. 1995;774:16–28.
36. Cellai I, Di Stasi V, Comeglio P, et al. Insight on the intracrinology of menopause: androgen production within the human vagina. Endocrinology. 2020;162:bqaa219. Epub ahead of print.
37. Phelan N, O'Connor A, Kyaw-Tun T, et al. Lipoprotein subclass patterns in women with polycystic ovary syndrome (PCOS) compared with equally insulin-resistant women without PCOS. J Clin Endocrinol Metab. 2010;95:3933.
38. Berneis K, Rizzo M, Lazzarini V, et al. Atherogenic lipoprotein phenotype and low-density lipoproteins size and subclasses in women with polycystic ovary syndrome. J Clin Endocrinol Metab. 2007;92:186.
39. Zhao D, Guallar E, Ouyang P, et al. Endogenous sex hormones and incident cardiovascular disease in post-menopausal women. J Am Coll Cardiol. 2018;71(22):2555–66.
40. Montalcini T, Migliaccio V, Ferro Y, Gazzaruso C, Pujia A. Androgens for postmenopausal women's health? Endocrine. 2012;42:514–20.
41. Patel SM, Ratcliffe SJ, Reilly MP, et al. Higher serum testosterone concentration in older women is associated with insulin resistance, metabolic syndrome, and cardiovascular disease. J Clin Endocrinol Metab. 2009;94:4776–84.
42. Maturana MA, Breda V, Lhullier F, Spritzer PM. Relationship between endogenous testosterone and cardiovascular risk in early postmenopausal women. Metabolism. 2008;57:961–5.
43. Laughlin GA, Goodell V, Barrett-Connor E. Extremes of endogenous testosterone are associated with increased risk of incident coronary events in older women. J Clin Endocrinol Metab. 2010;95(2):740–7.
44. Jones RD, High Jones T, Channer KS. The influence of testosterone upon vascular reactivity. Eur J Endocrinol. 2004;151(1):29–37.
45. Krapf JM, Simon JA. The role of testosterone in the management of hypoactive sexual desire disorder in postmenopausal women. Maturitas. 2009;63:213–9.

46. Miller KK, Sesmilo G, Schiller A, Schoenfeld D, Burton S, Klibanski A. Androgen deficiency in women with hypopituitarism. J Clin Endocrinol Metab. 2001;86(2):561–7.
47. Soman M, Huang LC, Cai WH, et al. Serum androgen profiles in women with premature ovarian insufficiency: a systematic review and meta-analysis. Menopause. 2019;26(1):78–93.
48. Gordon CM, Grace E, Emans SJ, et al. Effects of oral dehydroepiandrosterone on bone density in young women with anorexia nervosa: a randomized trial. J Clin Endocrinol Metab. 2002;87(11):4935–41.
49. Nordmark G, Bengtsson C, Larsson A, Karlsson FA, Sturfelt G, Rönnblom L. Effects of dehydroepiandrosterone supplement on health-related quality of life in glucocorticoid treated female patients with systemic lupus erythematosus. Autoimmunity. 2005;38:531–40.
50. Arlt W, Justl HG, Callies F, et al. Oral dehydroepiandrosterone for adrenal androgen replacement: pharmacokinetics and peripheral conversion to androgens and estrogens in young healthy females after dexamethasone suppression. J Clin Endocrinol Metab. 1998;83:1928–34.
51. Huang JS, Wilkie SJ, Dolan S, et al. Reduced testosterone levels in human immunodeficiency virus-infected women with weight loss and low weight. Clin Infect Dis. 2003;36:499–506.
52. Sinha-Hikim I, Arver S, Beall G, et al. The use of a sensitive equilibrium dialysis method for the measurement of free testosterone levels in healthy, cycling women and in human immunodeficiency virus-infected women. J Clin Endocrinol Metab. 1998;83:1312–8.
53. Wang C, Catlin D, Demers L, Borislav S, Swerdloff R. Measurement of total serum testosterone in adult men: comparison of current laboratory methods versus liquid chromatography tandem mass spectrometry. J Clin Endocrinol Metab. 2004;89(2):534–43.
54. Harwood DT, Handelsman DJ. Development and validation of a sensitive liquid chromatography-tandem mass spectrometry assay to simultaneously measure androgens and estrogens in serum without derivatization. Clin Chim Acta. 2009;409:78–84.
55. Demers LM. Androgen deficiency in women; role of accurate testosterone measurements. Maturitas. 2010;67(1):39–45.
56. Miller KK. Androgen deficiency in women. J Clin Endocrinol Metab. 2001;86(6):2395–401.
57. Miller KK, Rosner W, Lee H, et al. Measurement of free testosterone in normal women and women with androgen deficiency: comparison of methods. J Clin Endocrinol Metab. 2004;89(2):525–33.
58. Davis SR, Baber R, Panay N, et al. Global Consensus Position Statement on the use of testosterone therapy for women. J Clin Endocrinol Metab. 2019;104(10):4660–6.
59. Rosner W, Vesper H. Toward excellence in testosterone testing: a consensus statement. J Clin Endocrinol Metab. 2010;95:4542–8.
60. Rosen R, Brown C, Heiman J, et al. The Female Sexual Function Index (FSFI): a multidimensional self-report instrument for the assessment of female sexual function. J Sex Marital Ther. 2000;26:191–208.
61. Simon J, Braunstein G, Nachtigall L, et al. Testosterone patch increases sexual activity and desire in surgically menopausal women with hypoactive sexual desire disorder. J Clin Endocrinol Metab. 2005;90:5226–33.
62. Davis SR, van der Mooren MJ, van Lunsen RH, et al. Efficacy and safety of a testosterone patch for the treatment of hypoactive sexual desire disorder in surgically menopausal women: a randomized, placebo-controlled trial. Menopause. 2006;13:387–96.
63. Panay N, Al-Azzawi F, Bouchard C, et al. Testosterone treatment of HSDD in naturally menopausal women: the ADORE study. Climacteric J. 2010;13:121–31.
64. Achilli C, Pundir J, Ramanathan P, Sabatini L, Hamoda H, Panay N. Efficacy and safety of transdermal testosterone in postmenopausal women with hypoactive sexual desire disorder: a systematic review and meta-analysis. Fertil Steril. 2017;107(2):475–482 e415.
65. Buster JE, Kingsberg SA, Aguirre O, et al. Testosterone patch for low sexual desire in surgically menopausal women: a randomized trial. Obstet Gynecol. 2005;105:944–52.
66. Shifren JL, Davis SR, Moreau M, et al. Testosterone patch for the treatment of hypoactive sexual desire disorder in naturally menopausal women: results from the INTIMATE NM1 study. Menopause. 2006;13(5):770–9.

67. Braunstein GD, Sundwall DA, Katz M, et al. Safety and efficacy of a testosterone patch for the treatment of hypoactive sexual desire disorder in surgically menopausal women: a randomized, placebo-controlled trial. Arch Intern Med. 2005;165(14):1582–9.
68. Islam RM, Bell RJ, Green S, Page MJ, Davis SR. Safety and efficacy of testosterone for women: a systematic review and meta-analysis of randomised controlled trial data. Lancet Diabetes Endocrinol. 2019;7(10):754–66.
69. Withdrawal assessment report for Intrinsa Procedure No. EMEA/H/C/000634/II/0013.
70. Goldstat R, Briganti E, Tran J, Wolfe R, Davis SR. Transdermal testosterone therapy improves well-being, mood, and sexual function in premenopausal women. Menopause. 2003;10:390–8.
71. Dias RS, Kerr-Corrêa F, Moreno RA, et al. Efficacy of hormone therapy with and without methyltestosterone augmentation of venlafaxine in the treatment of postmenopausal depression: a double-blind controlled pilot study. Menopause. 2006;13:202–11.
72. Miller KK, Perlis RH, Papakostas GI, et al. Low-dose transdermal testosterone augmentation therapy improves depression severity in women. CNS Spectr. 2009;14:688–94.
73. Elraiyah T, Sonbol MB, Wang Z, et al. Clinical review: the benefits and harms of systemic testosterone therapy in postmenopausal women with normal adrenal function: a systematic review and meta-analysis. J Clin Endocrinol Metab. 2014;99:3543.
74. Somboonporn W, Davis S, Seif MW, Bell R. Testosterone for peri- and postmenopausal women. Cochrane Database Syst Rev. 2005;(4):CD004509.
75. Ling S, Komesaroff PA, Sudhir K. Cardiovascular physiology of androgens and androgen testosterone therapy in postmenopausal women. Endocr Metab Immune Disord Drug Targets. 2009;9(1):29–37.
76. Barrett-Connor E, Young R, Notelovitz M, et al. A two-year, double-blind comparison of estrogen-androgen and conjugated estrogens in surgically menopausal women. Effects on bone mineral density, symptoms and lipid profiles. J Reprod Med. 1999;44:1012–20.
77. Chiuve SE, Martin LA, Campos H, Sacks FM. Effect of the combination of methyltestosterone and esterified estrogens compared with esterified estrogens alone on apolipoprotein CIII and other apolipoproteins in very low density, low density, and high density lipoproteins in surgically postmenopausal women. J Clin Endocrinol Metab. 2004;89:2207–13.
78. Wagner JD, Zhang L, Williams JK, et al. Esterified estrogens with and without methyltestosterone decrease arterial LDL metabolism in cynomolgus monkeys. Arterioscler Thromb Vasc Biol. 1996;16:1473–80.
79. Davis SR, McCloud P, Strauss BJ, Burger H. Testosterone enhances estradiol's effects on postmenopausal bone density and sexuality. Maturitas. 1995;21:227–36.
80. Davis SR, Moreau M, Kroll R, et al. Testosterone for low libido in postmenopausal women not taking estrogen. N Engl J Med. 2008;359:2005–17.
81. Davis S, Papalia MA, Norman RJ, et al. Safety and efficacy of a testosterone metered-dose transdermal spray for treating decreased sexual satisfaction in premenopausal women: a randomized trial. Ann Intern Med. 2008;148:569–77.
82. Spoletini I, Vitale C, Pelliccia F, et al. Androgens and cardiovascular disease in postmenopausal women: a systematic review. Climacteric. 2014;17(6):625–35.
83. Penotti M, Sironi L, Cannata L, et al. Effects of androgen supplementation of hormone replacement therapy on the vascular reactivity of cerebral arteries. Fertil Steril. 2001;76:235–40.
84. Jayasena CN, Alkaabi FM, Liebers CS, Handley T, Franks S, Dhillo WS. A systematic review of randomized controlled trials investigating the efficacy and safety of testosterone therapy for female sexual dysfunction in postmenopausal women. Clin Endocrinol (Oxf). 2019;90(3):391–414.
85. Nachtigall L, Casson P, Lucas J, Schofield V, Melson C, Simon JA. Safety and tolerability of testosterone patch therapy for up to 4 years in surgically menopausal women receiving oral or transdermal oestrogen. Gynecol Endocrinol. 2011;27(1):39–48.

86. Flöter A, Nathorst-böös J, Carlström K, Ohlsson C, Ringertz H, von Schoultz B. Effects of combined estrogen/testosterone therapy on bone and body composition in oophorectomized women. Gynecol Endocrinol. 2005;20(3):155–60.
87. Huang G, Tang E, Aakil A, et al. Testosterone dose-response relationships with cardiovascular risk markers in androgen-deficient women: a randomized, placebo-controlled trial. J Clin Endocrinol Metab. 2014;99(7):1287–93.
88. Khosla S, Riggs BL, Robb RA, et al. Relationship of volumetric bone density and structural parameters at different skeletal sites to sex steroid levels in women. J Clin Endocrinol Metab. 2005;90:5096–103.
89. Miller KK, Biller BM, Beauregard C, et al. Effects of testosterone replacement in androgen-deficient women with hypopituitarism: a randomized, double-blind, placebo-controlled study. J Clin Endocrinol Metab. 2006;91:1683–90.
90. Watts NB, Notelovitz M, Timmons MC, Addison WA, Wiita B, Downey LJ. Comparison of oral estrogens and estrogens plus androgen on bone mineral density, menopausal symptoms, and lipid- lipoprotein profiles in surgical menopause. Obstet Gynecol. 1995;85:529–37.
91. Garnett T, Studd J, Watson N, Savvas M, Leather A. The effects of plasma estradiol levels on increases in vertebral and femoral bone density following therapy with estradiol and estradiol with testosterone implants. Obstet Gynecol. 1992;79:968–72.
92. Miller BE, De Souza MJ, Slade K, Luciano AA. Sublingual administration of micronized estradiol and progesterone, with and without micronized testosterone: effect on biochemical markers of bone metabolism and bone mineral density. Menopause. 2000;7:318–26.
93. Simon JA, Goldstein I, Kim NN, et al. The role of androgens in the treatment of genitourinary syndrome of menopause (GSM): International Society for the Study of Women's sexual health (ISSWSH) expert consensus panel review. Menopause. 2018;25:837–47.
94. Bell RJ, Rizvi F, Islam RM, et al. A systematic review of intravaginal testosterone for the treatment of vulvovaginal atrophy. Menopause. 2018;25:704–9.
95. Maseroli E, Vignozzi L. Testosterone and vaginal function. Sex Med Rev. 2020;8(3):379–92.
96. Raghunandan C, Agrawal S, Dubey P, Choudhury M, Jain A. A comparative study of the effects of local estrogen with or without local testosterone on vulvovaginal and sexual dysfunction in post- menopausal women. J Sex Med. 2010;7:1284–90.
97. Witherby S, Johnson J, Demers L, et al. Topical testosterone for breast cancer patients with vaginal atrophy related to aromatase inhibitors: a phase I/II study. Oncologist. 2011;16:424–31.
98. Labrie F, Archer D, Bouchard C, et al. Effect of intravaginal dehydroepiandrosterone (Prasterone) on libido and sexual dysfunction in postmenopausal women. Menopause. 2009;16:923–31.
99. Labrie F, Archer D, Bouchard C, et al. Lack of influence of dyspareunia on the beneficial effect of intravaginal prasterone (dehydroepiandrosterone, DHEA) on sexual dysfunction in postmenopausal women. J Sex Med. 2014;11:1766–85.
100. Labrie F, Archer DF, Koltun W, et al. Efficacy of intravaginal dehydroepiandrosterone (DHEA) on moderate to severe dyspareunia and vaginal dryness, symptoms of vulvovaginal atrophy, and of the genitourinary syndrome of menopause. Menopause. 2018;25:1339–53.
101. European Medicines Agency. Intrarosa: European public assessment report. 2017. http://www.ema.europa.eu. Accessed 20 June 2019.
102. Shifren JL, Braunstein GD, Simon JA, et al. Transdermal testosterone treatment in women with impaired sexual function after oophorectomy. N Engl J Med. 2000;343:682–8.
103. Somboonporn W, Davis S. Testosterone effects on the breast: implications for testosterone therapy for women. Endocr Rev. 2004;25:374–88.
104. Key TJ, Appleby PN, Reeves GK, Endogenous Hormones and Breast Cancer Collaborative Group, et al. Sex hormones and risk of breast cancer in premenopausal women: a collaborative reanalysis of individual participant data from seven prospective studies. Lancet Oncol. 2013;14:1009–19.
105. Key TJ, Appleby PN, Reeves GK, Endogenous Hormones and Breast Cancer Collaborative Group, et al. Steroid hormone measurements from different types of assays in relation to

body mass index and breast cancer risk in postmenopausal women: reanalysis of 18 prospective studies. Steroids. 2015;99:49–55.
106. Baglietto L, Severi G, English DR, et al. Circulating steroid hormone levels and risk of breast cancer for postmenopausal women. Cancer Epidemiol Biomarkers Prev. 2010;19:492–502.
107. Sieri S, Krogh V, Bolelli G, et al. Sex hormone levels, breast cancer risk, and cancer receptor status in postmenopausal women: the ORDET cohort. Cancer Epidemiol Biomarkers Prev. 2009;18:169–76.
108. Wang B, Mi M, Wang J, et al. Does the increase of endogenous steroid hormone levels also affect breast cancer risk in Chinese women? A case-control study in Chongqing, China. Int J Cancer. 2009;124:1892–9.
109. Davis SR, Hirschberg AL, Wagner LK, Lodhi I, von Schoultz B. The effect of transdermal testosterone on mammographic density in postmenopausal women not receiving systemic estrogen therapy. J Clin Endocrinol Metab. 2009;94:4907–13.
110. Tamimi RM, Hankinson SE, Chen WY, Rosner B, Colditz GA. Combined estrogen and testosterone use and risk of breast cancer in postmenopausal women. Arch Intern Med. 2006;166:1483–9.
111. Jick SS, Hagberg KW, Kaye JA, Jick H. Postmenopausal estrogen-containing hormone therapy and the risk of breast cancer. Obstet Gynecol. 2009;113:74–80.
112. Dimitrakakis C, Jones RA, Liu A, Bondy CA. Breast cancer incidence in postmenopausal women using testosterone in addition to usual hormone therapy. Menopause. 2004;11:531–5.
113. Davis SR, Wolfe R, Farrugia H, Ferdinand A, Bell RJ. The incidence of invasive breast cancer among women prescribed testosterone for low libido. J Sex Med. 2009;6:1850–6.
114. Glaser RL, York AE, Dimitrakakis C. Incidence of invasive breast cancer in women treated with testosterone implants: a prospective 10-year cohort study. BMC Cancer. 2019;19(1):1271.
115. Agency EM. Withdrawal assessment report for Intrinsa. London, UK; 2010.
116. Maia H Jr, Maltez A, Fahel P, Athayde C, Coutinho E. Detection of testosterone and estrogen receptors in the postmenopausal endometrium. Maturitas. 2001;38:179–88.
117. Filho AM, Barbosa IC, Maia H Jr, Genes CC, Coutinho EM. Effects of subdermal implants of estradiol and testosterone on the endometrium of postmenopausal women. Gynecol Endocrinol. 2007;23:511–7.
118. Laumann E, Paik A, Rosen RC. Sexual dysfunction in the United States: prevalence and predictors. JAMA. 1999;281:531–44.
119. Clayton A, Goldstein I, Kim NN, Althof SE, Faubion SS, Faught BM, Parish SJ, Simon J, Vignozzi L, Christiansen K, Davis SR, Freedman MA, Kingsberg SA, Kirana P-S, Larkin L, McCabe M, Sadovsky R. The International Society for the Study of Women's Sexual Health process of care for management of hypoactive sexual desire disorder in women. Mayo Clin Proc. 2018;93(4):467–87.
120. ADDYI (flibanserin) [package insert]. Bridgewater, NJ: Sprout Pharmaceuticals; 2016.
121. Katz M, DeRogatis LR, Ackerman R, BEGONIA Trial Investigators, et al. Efficacy of flibanserin in women with hypoactive sexual desire disorder: results from the BEGONIA trial. J Sex Med. 2013;10(7):1807–15.
122. Thorp J, Simon J, Dattani D, DAISY Trial Investigators, et al. Treatment of hypoactive sexual desire disorder in premenopausal women: efficacy of flibanserin in the DAISY study. J Sex Med. 2012;9(3):793–804.
123. Derogatis LR, Komer L, Katz M, VIOLET Trial Investigators, et al. Treatment of hypoactive sexual desire disorder in pre- menopausal women: efficacy of flibanserin in the VIOLET study. J Sex Med. 2012;9(4):1074–85.
124. Shifren JL, Davis SR. Androgens in postmenopausal women: a review. Menopause. 2017;24(8):970–9.
125. Scheffers CS, Armstrong S, Cantineau AE, et al. Dehydroepiandrosterone for women in the peri- or postmenopausal phase. Cochrane Database Syst Rev. 2015;1:CD011066.
126. Leder BZ, Leblanc KM, Longcope C, et al. Effects of oral androstenedione administration on serum testosterone and estradiol levels in postmenopausal women. J Clin Endocrinol Metab. 2002;87:5449.

Chapter 9
Testosterone in Transgender Population

Carlotta Cocchetti and Alessandra Daphne Fisher

9.1 Introduction

Gender incongruence (GI) is defined by a marked and persistent incongruence between an individual's experienced gender and the assigned one at birth [1]. In cases where the condition leads to clinically significant distress or impairment in social, occupational, or other important areas of functioning, it is referred to as gender dysphoria (GD) [2]. Individuals whose gender identity does not completely and/or permanently match their sex characteristics may describe themselves as trans or transgender [2]. In particular, we use the term transgender men for those assigned female at birth who identify as men and transgender women for those assigned males who identify as women.

GI/GD represents a dimensional phenomenon that can occur with different degrees of intensity, of which the most extreme form is accompanied by the desire for gender affirming treatment, including hormonal treatment and/or surgical interventions.

Health care providers (HCPs) dealing with transgender health care should openly ask for the individual gender experience of the person seeking treatment and explore desired hormonal treatment effects, in order to guarantee an individualized approach [3]. If mental health concerns are identified at the time of initial evaluation, they should be reasonably well controlled before starting GAHT [4]. In considering GAHT in individuals with mental health concerns, it is relevant to note that hormonal treatment has been associated with an improved quality of life and a decrease in psychiatric morbidities, such as anxiety, depression, and suicide risk [5–8].

Furthermore, before the start of GAHT, transgender individuals should be screened by hormone-providing professionals for medical conditions that can be

C. Cocchetti · A. D. Fisher (✉)
Andrology, Women's Endocrinology and Gender Incongruence Unit, Careggi University Hospital, Florence, Italy
e-mail: fishera@aou-careggi.toscana.it

© Springer Nature Switzerland AG 2021
J. P. Mulhall et al. (eds.), *Controversies in Testosterone Deficiency*,
https://doi.org/10.1007/978-3-030-77111-9_9

exacerbated by hormone depletion and treatment with sex hormones of the affirmed gender. The clinical evaluation should include an exhaustive medical history, including thromboembolic diseases, arterial hypertension, polycythaemia and sleep apnoea [9]. In this phase, expected results and possible adverse effects must be discussed by the clinicians, as well as fertility issues. In fact, fertility preservation options should be discussed by the HCP with the patient early in the transition process and with the endocrinologist before starting GAHT [3].

9.2   Gender Affirming Hormones in Transgender Men

The classical main goals of GAHT are to reduce endogenous sex hormone levels, and thus reduce the secondary sex characteristics of the individual's assigned gender, and to replace endogenous sex hormone levels consistent with the individual's gender identity. Since gender identity is a continuum that exists between male and female, transgender men may desire different outcomes from GAHT, ranging from an androgynous presentation to maximal virilization. Ideally, the ultimate GAHT regimen should integrate several factors, including the patients' objectives, risk-to-benefit ratio and social/economic considerations [4, 10]. However, to date there are no evidence-based recommendations for personalized therapies in non-binary individuals.

Hormonal treatment in transgender men consists of different testosterone formulations, generally administered intramuscularly, subcutaneously, or transdermal. Regimen of GAHT in transgender men follows similar principles of hormonal therapies for male hypogonadism, with the aim to achieve cisgender male reference ranges for serum testosterone levels (typically from 300 to 1000 ng/dL) [9]. Sustained supraphysiologic levels of testosterone are associated with increased risks of adverse reactions and should be avoided. GAHT with testosterone needs to be continued after ovariectomy, in order to maintain virilization and to avoid hypogonadism symptoms.

Regarding available testosterone formulations, injectable testosterone esters represent the most commonly prescribed in transgender men, used in dosages of 200–250 mg intramuscularly or subcutaneously every 2 or 3 weeks, or lower doses weekly [9]. However, these formulations require frequent injections resulting in peaks and troughs in testosterone levels that may have consequences on mood and erythrocytosis [11]. Another formulation commonly used by clinicians is represented by long-acting testosterone undecanoate 750–1000 mg, administered intramuscularly every 10–12 weeks, after an initial loading dose at baseline and after 4–6 weeks [9]. Disadvantages with the longer duration formulations may include cost, the inability to self-administer, the large injection volume and a small risk of pulmonary microembolism. Other options include topical gel 1.62–2% (25–100 mg/d), transdermal patches (2.5–10 mg/d), and intransal or buccal formulations. Oral testosterone undecanoate is a rarely used option for GAHT because of high absorption variability leading to variable testosterone concentrations. Additionally, it is not available in many locations, such as the United States. Although the majority of research on GAHT in transgender men has used long-acting intramuscular testosterone undecanoate or topical gels, other modalities appear to be comparable regarding efficacy, safety, and patient satisfaction [12].

Testosterone treatment is generally considered safe in the short term and mid-term, based on existing data. However, the literature specific to transgender populations is limited, with a paucity of high-quality, long-term data available. This lack is partially ascribable to unique challenges with transgender cohorts, including the unethical nature of randomized studies, differing end goals, and smaller numbers overall for recruitment.

9.3 Desirable Effects

In transgender men, testosterone results in progressive virilization, leading to deepening of the voice, development/coarsening of facial and body hair in a male pattern, increased muscle mass, clitoromegaly and cessation of menses. As the body changes increasingly align with the perceived gender identity, decrease in body uneasiness is observed in many individuals [7].

9.3.1 Voice

Similar to the effects of increased testosterone levels during pubertal development, testosterone treatment leads to hypertrophy of muscle cells with a reduction of surrounding fat cells at the level of the larynx, inducing a lowering of the pitch of the voice [13]. Generally, virilizing effects on the voice of birth-assigned women are observed at serum testosterone levels ≥150 µg/dL, while prolonged exposure to concentrations >200 µg/dL induces irreversible changes, usually occurring during the first 3 months of testosterone treatment [14]. In the majority (90%) of transmen, voice cannot be distinguished from those of natal men [15, 16]. Additionally, a voice perceived as male is generally associated with higher well-being compared with those with less gender-congruent voices [17].

9.3.2 Dermatologic Effects

One of the most important effects of testosterone therapy is the development of facial and body hair, since the pilosebaceous unit of the skin expresses both androgen and oestrogen receptors. An increase of body and facial hair – assessed through the Ferriman-Gallwey score – begins during the first year of testosterone treatment, although Ferriman-Gallwey scores are still lower compared with cisgender men [18]. Further increases of body and facial hair growth continue to occur beyond one year, although long-term data are lacking [19].

9.3.3 Reproductive Organs

Testosterone treatment induces changes in serum concentrations of reproductive and pituitary hormones, including increased testosterone and decreased oestrogen and sex hormone-binding globulin [12, 20]. Regarding luteinizing hormone and follicle-stimulating hormone, most studies have shown that testosterone therapy is associated with reduced or totally suppressed levels of gonadotropins [19]. Nakamura et al. [21] reported a cessation of menstruation – usually desired – in a high percentage (86–97%) of transgender men by 6 months of testosterone enanthate treatment. In another study [12], time to amenorrhoea ranged from 30 to 41 weeks, with all participants reporting amenorrhoea by 1 year of testosterone treatment.

Another desired effect of gender affirming hormonal treatment is represented by clitoral enlargement. This effect becomes apparent after only 3 months of testosterone therapy (>60%, mean clitoral length after 3 months: 3.19 ± 0.54 cm), but the clitoris continues to grow during testosterone administration (mean length after 2 years: 3.83 ± 0.42 cm) [7]. However, clitoris enlargement is often associated with pain. In a 1-year prospective study including transgender men under testosterone undecanoate, clitoral pain was reported in 20% of participants and reached a peak after 6 months of treatment [22].

9.3.4 Sexual Well-Being

The relationship between sexual desire and circulating levels of testosterone in cis-gender men is well established in the literature [23, 24]. However, this relationship is more complex in cisgender women. In this population, testosterone administration in moderate doses results in increased sexual desire and satisfaction, while high-dose administration seems to have a lower efficacy, probably because of undesirable clinical effects of hyperandrogenism [25]. In transgender men, the literature concerning the impact of hormonal treatment before gender affirming surgery is scarce. However, an increase in sexual desire is reported in transmen after the start of testosterone treatment [26]. Additionally, Costantino and colleagues [24] described an increase in sexual desire, masturbation, sexual fantasies, and arousal after 1 year of testosterone administration. Furthermore, in transgender men, GAHT is associated with a reduction of sexually related distress across time, possibly due to improved congruence between the body and perceived gender [27].

9.3.5 Body Composition

Testosterone treatment induces body composition changes towards those of natal men, who on average have a more representative lean mass than natal women. Several studies reported an increase of bodyweight, lean mass, and body mass index

(BMI) during testosterone treatment [28–32]. Furthermore, some of them showed a decrease in fat mass of 2.3–4.0 kg [30, 31].

A prospective study by Van Caenegem and colleagues described an increased grip strength, as well as an increased cross-sectional area of the forearm and calf muscles, after 1-yr of testosterone undecanoate treatment [32].

9.4   Side Effects

9.4.1   Dermatologic Effects

The pilosebaceous unit is a well-known androgen target tissue, in which testosterone and the active metabolite dihydrotestosterone play a central role in stimulation of sebaceous gland growth and differentiation [33, 34]. This leads not only to desired dermatological effects of testosterone treatment, such as development of facial and body hair, but also to dermatological side effects, such as acne and androgenetic alopecia in transgender men who are genetically predisposed.

Testosterone treatment leads to an increase in acne at the face and back after 4 months, with a peak severity after 6 months [19]. However, most patients develop only mild acne, which usually decreases by 12 months of treatment and has been reported to resolve longer term (10-year follow-up) [19].

Although acne develops within months after starting GAHT, androgenetic alopecia represents a longer-term side effect of testosterone administration. Previous studies reported incidence rates of androgenetic alopecia – based on the Norwood-Hamilton classification system – of 17% after 1 year of treatment and moderate to severe androgenetic alopecia of 31% after 10 years [19]. Although alopecia is considered a side effect of testosterone use, it may be desirable for some transgender men, since it is considered a typical masculine feature.

9.4.2   Reproductive Organs

Testosterone treatment induces morphological changes in the vagina, endometrium and ovaries. Several studies reported a thinner vaginal epithelium, with a loss of the intermediate and superficial layers, and other microstructural changes, such as a loss of intracytoplasmic glycogen, reduced expression of oestrogen receptor α and β and reduced cellular proliferation [35]. These changes are associated with decreased vaginal lubrication, which can result in vaginal dryness or itching and painful penetration [36].

With regard to the ovaries, GAHT is associated with stromal hyperplasia, increased volume and a histological pattern similar to that reported in patients with polycystic ovary syndrome [37].

Studies evaluating endometrial changes have reported inconsistent results, with some describing a proliferative pattern and others an atrophic one [37, 38].

9.4.3 Cardiovascular Safety

The cardiovascular impact of testosterone treatment in transgender men remains poorly understood and controversial. Testosterone may exert its effects through several mechanisms, including changes in insulin sensitivity, lipid profile, blood pressure, red cell count and platelet aggregation [39]. Testosterone treatment in transgender men impacts several independent cardiac risk factors, such as lipid profile, blood pressure and haematocrit level. Despite these alterations, the actual impact on cardiovascular events remains understudied, with no evidence for increased risks in the short and medium terms. Elamin and colleagues [40] conducted a systematic review of the literature and concluded that the level of evidence was too low to provide an interpretation for the risk of testosterone therapy on cardiovascular morbidity and mortality in transgender men.

The literature regarding the impact of hormonal treatment on blood pressure has also demonstrated conflicting results. Most studies reported an increase in systolic blood pressure of 4–12 mmHg without any significant changes in diastolic blood pressure after 1 year of testosterone treatment [22, 29, 30]. Another prospective study reported an increase in both systolic and diastolic blood pressure in adolescent transgender men after 2 years of hormonal treatment [41]. In contrast, two prospective studies observed no changes in systolic or diastolic blood pressure in adult transgender men after the start of testosterone treatment [42, 43].

Given these discrepant reports, the impact of testosterone therapy on blood pressure, and in turn on cardiovascular risk long term, is unknown.

Research on the impact of testosterone treatment on lipid profiles remains limited. The lipid parameter most consistently affected by testosterone treatment in transgender men is HDL cholesterol. Several studies reported a decrease of 4–13 mg/dL during the first year of testosterone treatment, independent of formulation [29–31, 44–47]. However, since it is possible that HDL metabolism is more predictive of atherogenicity than circulating HDL, further research is required to determine the clinical relevance of these findings. Some data have suggested increased atherogenicity in transgender men- related to increased triglyceride levels and decreased HDL2 and HDL3 levels-, while others have demonstrated decreased atherogenicity [47, 48]. Regarding LDL levels, two prospective studies reported a decrease after 12–18 months of testosterone undecanoate [49, 50], while others described an increase or no changes in LDL levels [22, 43]. Findings from different studies [22, 30, 31] have also shown an increase in triglycerides during the first 2 years with topical and intramuscular testosterone administration.

In a recent systematic review and meta-analysis including 29 studies, Maraka and colleagues concluded that testosterone administration was associated with an increase in LDL and triglycerides levels and a decrease in HDL in transgender men, although the quality of evidence remains low [51].

Testosterone therapy does not appear to affect fasting serum glucose or insulin sensitivity in transgender men, which is further supported by hyperinsulinemic-euglycemic clamp studies [41, 45, 52, 53].

Regarding metabolic cytokines, testosterone treatment may reverse the observed sexual dimorphism in adiponectin and leptin levels, probably directly regulating their secretion from adipose tissues. Two prospective studies reported a decrease in both leptin and adiponectin levels during testosterone therapy in transgender men [28, 54].

All testosterone formulations lead to increases in haemoglobin (>4.9–12.5% range) and haematocrit (>4.4–17.6% range) levels, with the most marked increase occurring during the first 3 months of hormonal treatment. Haematocrit then appears to stabilize after the first year of treatment [11, 49, 50]. Clinically significant erythrocytosis is rare and the impact of haematocrit levels on cardiovascular and thrombotic risk is not well studied.

Only one study has investigated the impact of testosterone administration in transgender men on coagulation profiles and reported an overall antithrombotic effect with testosterone due to lower activated protein C resistance [55]. Similarly, testosterone treatment is not associated with an increased incidence of venous thromboembolism in transgender men [56, 57].

Regarding cardiovascular events, Wierckx and colleagues [58] compared the prevalence of cardiovascular disease between 138 transgender men using testosterone for an average of 9 years and age-matched, cisgender women and found no differences in myocardial infarction or cerebrovascular disease rates.

In summary, data on cardiovascular safety of GAHT are limited and contradictory. For this reason, further research is needed, especially in older transgender men, rather than in young individuals who are at low risk of cardiovascular events.

9.4.4   Hepatologic and Renal Safety

In the past, hepatotoxicity was a significant issue with orally administered 17-alkylated testosterone. However, since this compound is no longer recommended, serious hepatic toxicity is rare with contemporary testosterone therapies [9, 59, 60].

Two prospective studies reported no significant increase in liver enzymes in transgender men during gender affirming hormonal treatment [20, 50]. Another prospective study from Wierckx and colleagues [22] reported a significant increase of liver enzymes after 1 year of testosterone treatment. However, only 1.9% of transgender men had liver enzyme values exceeding twice the upper limit of normal according to female ranges and none exceeding twice the upper limit of normal according to male reference ranges.

Regarding kidney function, two prospective studies described an increase in creatinine levels after 1 year of testosterone treatment [22, 61]. However, transgender men receiving testosterone treatment have similar creatinine concentrations to transgender women at baseline, suggesting that creatinine changes may simply be reflective of body changes that are expected to occur with testosterone therapy rather than being considered as a pathological change [61].

9.4.5 Bone Health

One of the goals of testosterone treatment in transgender men is to reduce oestradiol concentrations, which may hypothetically lead to decreased bone mineral density (BMD). However, a recent meta-analysis [62] reported similar BMD in cisgender women and transgender men before testosterone treatment, with no decreases in BMD after testosterone initiation. Van Caenegem and colleagues [63] described an increased radial cortical bone size and decreased cortical volumetric BMD at the radius and tibia in transgender men receiving testosterone treatment when compared to age-matched natal women. The explanation for these observations may relate to the fact that testosterone is readily converted to oestrogen via the aromatase enzyme and therefore maintains sufficient oestrogen levels. In addition, increased muscle mass leads to an increased mechanical load on the bone, which further stimulates bone formation. Indeed, the previously cited study observed a positive correlation between muscle mass, strength and trabecular and cortical parameters and bone size [63]. As with other BMD literature, there is a lack of data on osteoporotic fracture risk in transgender men, with the only published study demonstrating no fractures after 12 months of follow-up [22]. It is noteworthy that in cases where the patient undergoes ovariectomy, testosterone therapy is fundamental to reduce oestrogen-deprivation-related bone loss. Indeed, bone loss has been described after ovariectomy in transgender men who stopped or were not compliant with hormonal treatment [64–66].

9.4.6 Oncological Risk

Oncological risk represents one of the most critical issues in transgender health care. Currently, prospective studies with adequate sample size and follow-up duration are lacking. This is extremely critical considering that transgender population is more frequently exposed to cancer risk factors, such as smoking, obesity and drug abuse. Additionally, given the discomfort that transgender men experience accessing gynaecologic care, the rate of adequate cancer screening in this population is low.

Current guidelines recommend that transgender individuals adhere to similar screening protocols that are used for the general population according to birth-assigned sex if the organs are still present [9]. In addition, transgender men are recommended to undergo hysterectomy and oophorectomy to eliminate the risk of female reproductive tract disease and cancer [9]. To date, no large, representative, long-term, and prospective studies on cancer risk in transgender cohorts have been published, and available data are limited to case reports.

Testosterone treatment produces changes in the composition of breast tissue in transgender men, inducing a reduction of glandular tissue and an increase in fibrous connective tissue [37, 67]. In addition to histological changes, several cases of breast cancer have been reported in the literature [68–71]. A hypothetical mechanism may be from conversion of exogenous testosterone into oestradiol via aromatase, although no study has confirmed a causal relationship between testosterone and breast cancer in transgender men. Gooren and colleagues [72] reported a lower incidence of breast cancer in transgender men compared with cisgender women (5.9 vs 155 per 100.000 person-years). Similarly, a study of 148 transgender men who underwent mastectomy [73] found no invasive malignancy, although premalignant transformations were observed, including apocrine metaplasia (23.6%), lactational changes (2%), columnar cell changes (37.2%), usual ductal hyperplasia (27%), atypical ductal hyperplasia (3.4%).

Breast cancer might still occur after mastectomy developing in subareolar tissue, as reported in some cases [69, 71]. For this reason, the Endocrine Society recommends to perform subareolar and periareolar breast examinations annually after mastectomy [9]. In transgender men who did not undergo mastectomy, mammography is suggested for ongoing screening, according to the guidelines for birth-assigned sex.

Only three cases of cervical cancer have been described in transgender men receiving testosterone, although there is currently no known mechanistic association between testosterone and cervical cancer [74–76]. Rather, the presence of human papilloma virus (HPV) is a well-established risk for cervical cancer in birth-assigned women. Transgender men are less likely than cisgender women to engage in HPV prevention behaviours, and this may represent the main factor associated with cervical cancer risk in this population [77].

Although aromatization of testosterone to oestradiol in transgender men has been suggested as a risk factor for endometrial cancer [78], only one case of endometrial cancer has been described in the literature [74]. A retrospective examination of genital tract histopathology of 112 transgender men performed by Grynberg and colleagues [37] showed endometrial atrophy in 45% of cases and only one sample displayed endometrial hyperplasia with a small focus of adenocarcinoma.

Regarding ovarian cancer, only three cases are reported in transgender men in the literature [79, 80]. Grynberg and colleagues [37] reported no cases of ovarian cancer in a prospective cohort study of transgender men after 6 months of testosterone administration. It should be considered that many transgender men undergo hysteron-oophorectomy after 12 months of testosterone treatment, and this may limit the observation of ovarian cancer in this population.

9.4.7 Psychological Monitoring

Testosterone treatment is generally associated with an improved overall well-being in transgender men. As a population, transgender individuals report higher baseline levels of depression, anxiety and suicide risk compared to cisgender men [81–83]. However, after initiating GAHT, these levels decrease and are comparable to the general population [5, 7, 84]. Some of these improvements may be attributed to the effects of testosterone in the central nervous system, but a more likely explanation for mental health improvement is the reduction of gender dysphoria during GAHT.

The literature available on the association between testosterone and aggression in human is inconclusive, with a recent 1-year prospective study reporting no increased aggression or anger among transgender men receiving testosterone treatment [85]. However, based on historical studies, it is notable that current guidelines continue to warn about the potential aggression in transgender men receiving GAHT [4, 9].

9.4.8 Mortality

Data regarding mortality rates in transgender men are lacking, and the few studies that investigated this aspect have shown inconsistent results. Asscheman and colleagues [86] compared the mortality rates between 365 transgender men under testosterone treatment and the general population and found no differences. In a Swedish study [87] based one data coming from national death registry, a comparison between mortality rates of 133 transgender men and 1330 age- and birth sex-matched controls was performed. The authors found no differences in mortality rates during the first 10 years after gender affirming surgery. However, the curves diverged after 10 years, with transgender men showing higher mortality rates.

9.5   Monitoring During Testosterone Treatment

For patients receiving GAHT, the Endocrine Society recommends routine surveillance every 3 months during the first year and then one or two times per year, in order to monitor the virilizing effects and potential adverse reactions of testosterone [9]. Testosterone levels should be assessed every 3 months and should be maintained in the normal physiologic male range, thereby reducing the likelihood for adverse events resulting from supraphysiologic dosing. Since the most frequent adverse reaction is increased haematocrit levels, routine blood tests, including a haematocrit, should be carried out at baseline and every 3 months for the first year of testosterone treatment and then one to two times a year. In addition, clinicians are advised to monitor weight, blood pressure and lipid profile at regular intervals. Furthermore, screening for osteoporosis should be conducted in those individuals not compliant to testosterone treatment or with higher baseline risks for bone loss.

9.6   Conclusions

After few months of testosterone treatment, transgender men begin experiencing desirable, virilizing body changes. Generally, satisfaction rates are high and GAHT is very rarely regretted [9, 88–90]. Initial body changes with GAHT include an increase in body and facial hair, deepening of the voice, increased lean mass and decreased fat mass, and cessation of menstruation. At the same time, transgender men may experience an increase in sexual desire and a reduction of perceived stress, anxiety and depression. The development of acne represents the most common undesired effect and is usually limited to the first few months of treatment. Regarding blood parameters, the most frequent adverse effect is increased haematocrit, reaching levels comparable to biological males, while clinically significant erythrocytosis is rare.

To conclude, testosterone treatment appears to be safe in the short term. However, some critical issues remain, particularly relating to oncologic risk and cardiovascular safety. Given the limited data and clinical importance of these issues, further long-term studies with larger cohorts are mandated.

References

1. World Health Organisation. International classification of diseases 11th revision. Geneva: World Health Organisation; 2018. Available at: https://icd.who.int/. Accessed 27 Aug 2018.
2. American Psychiatric Association. Diagnostic and statistical manual of mental disorders (DSM-5). Arlington: American Psychiatric Publishers; 2013.
3. Arcelus J, De Vries ALC, Fisher AD, Nieder TO, Özer M, Motmans J. European Society for Sexual Medicine Position Statement "Assessment and hormonal management in adolescent and adult trans people, with attention for sexual function and satisfaction". J Sex Med. 2020;pii:S1743-6095(20)30045-X. https://doi.org/10.1016/j.jsxm.2020.01.012. [Epub ahead of print].
4. Coleman E, Bockting W, Botzer M, et al. Standards of care for the health of transsexual, transgender, and gender-nonconforming people, version 7. Int J Transgenderism. 2012;13:165–232.
5. Heylens G, Verroken C, De Cock S, et al. Effects of different steps in gender reassignment therapy on psychopathology: a prospective study of persons with a gender identity disorder. J Sex Med. 2014;11(1):119–26.
6. Fisher AD, Castellini G, Bandini E, et al. Cross-sex hormonal treatment and body uneasiness in individuals with gender dysphoria. J Sex Med. 2014;11(3):709–19.
7. Fisher AD, Castellini G, Ristori J, et al. Cross-sex hormone treatment and psychobiological changes in transsexual persons: two-year follow-up data. J Clin Endocrinol Metab. 2016;101(11):4260–9.
8. Gorin-Lazard A, Baumstarck K, Boyer L, et al. Is hormonal therapy associated with better quality of life in transsexuals? A cross-sectional study. J Sex Med. 2012;9(2):531–41.
9. Hembree WC, Cohen-Kettenis PT, Gooren L, et al. Endocrine treatment of gender-dysphoric/gender-incongruent persons: an Endocrine Society clinical practice guideline. J Clin Endocrinol Metab. 2017;102(11):3869–903.
10. Cocchetti C, Ristori J, Romani A, et al. Hormonal treatment strategies tailored to non-binary transgender individuals. J Clin Med. 2020;9(6):1609.
11. Defreyne J, Vantomme B, Van Caenegem E, et al. Prospective evaluation of hematocrit in gender-affirming hormone treatment: results from European Network for the Investigation of Gender Incongruence. Andrology. 2018;6:446–54.
12. Pelusi C, Costantino A, Martelli V, et al. Effects of three different testosterone formulations in female-to-male transsexual persons. J Sex Med. 2014;11:3002–11.
13. Evans S, Neave N, Wakelin D, et al. The relationship between testosterone and vocal frequencies in human males. Physiol Behav. 2008;93(4–5):783–8.

14. Bultynck C, Pas C, Defreyne J, et al. Self-perception of voice in transgender persons during cross-sex hormone therapy. Laryngoscope. 2017;127(12):2796–804.
15. Abitbol J, Abitbol P, Abitbol B. Sex hormones and the female voice. J Voice. 1999;13(3):424–46.
16. Cosyns M, Borsel J, Wierckx K, et al. Voice in female-to-male transsexual persons after long-term androgen therapy. Laryngoscope. 2014;124(6):1409–14.
17. Watt SO, Tskhay KO, Rule NO. Masculine voices predict well-being in female-tomale transgender individuals. Arch Sex Behav. 2017;47:963–72.
18. Giltay EJ, Gooren LJG. Effects of sex steroid deprivation/administration on hair growth and skin sebum production in transsexual males and females. J Clin Endocrinol Metab. 2000;85(8):2913–21.
19. Wierckx K, Van de Peer F, Verhaeghe E, et al. Short-and long-term clinical skin effects of testosterone treatment in trans men. J Sex Med. 2014;11(1):222–9.
20. Mueller A, Kiesewetter F, Binder H, et al. Long-term administration of testosterone undecanoate every 3 months for testosterone supplementation in female-to-male transsexuals. J Clin Endocrinol Metab. 2007;92(9):3470–5.
21. Nakamura A, Watanabe M, Sugimoto M, Sako T, Mahmood S, Kaku H, Nasu Y, Ishii K, Nagai A, Kumon H. Dose-response analysis of testosterone replacement therapy in patients with female to male gender identity disorder. Endocr J. 2013;60(3):275–81. Epub 2012 Oct 27.
22. Wierckx K, Van Caenegem E, Schreiner T, et al. Cross-sex hormone therapy in trans persons is safe and effective at short-time follow-up: results from the European network for the investigation of gender incongruence. J Sex Med. 2014;11:1999–2011.
23. Allan CA, Forbes EA, Strauss BJG, et al. Testosterone therapy increases sexual desire in ageing men with low-normal testosterone levels and symptoms of androgen deficiency. Int J Impot Res. 2008;20(4):396–401.
24. Costantino A, Cerpolini S, Alvisi S, et al. A prospective study on sexual function and mood in female-to-male transsexuals during testosterone administration and after sex reassignment surgery. J Sex Marital Ther. 2013;39(4):321–35.
25. Somboonporn W, Davis S, Seif MW, et al. Testosterone for peri- and postmenopausal women. Cochrane Database Syst Rev. 2005;(4):CD004509.
26. Wierckx K, Elaut E, Van Caenegem E, et al. Sexual desire in female-to-male transsexual persons: exploration of the role of testosterone administration. Eur J Endocrinol. 2011;165(2):331–7.
27. Ristori J, Cocchetti C, Castellini G, Pierdominici M, Cipriani A, Testi D, Gavazzi G, Mazzoli F, Mosconi M, Meriggiola MC, Cassioli E, Vignozzi L, Ricca V, Maggi M, Fisher AD. Hormonal treatment effect on sexual distress in transgender persons: 2-year follow-up data. J Sex Med. 2020;17(1):142–51.
28. Berra M, Armillotta F, D'Emidio L, et al. Testosterone decreases adiponectin levels in female to male transsexuals. Asian J Androl. 2006;8:725–9.
29. Colizzi M, Costa R, Scaramuzzi F, et al. Concomitant psychiatric problems and hormonal treatment induced metabolic syndrome in gender dysphoria individuals: a 2 year follow-up study. J Psychosom Res. 2015;78:399–406.
30. Mueller A, Haeberle L, Zollver H, et al. Effects of intramuscular testosterone undecanoate on body composition and bone mineral density in female-to-male transsexuals. J Sex Med. 2010;7:3190–8.
31. Quiros C, Patrascioiu I, Mora M, et al. Effect of cross-sex hormone treatment on cardiovascular risk factors in transsexual individuals. Experience in a specialized unit in Catalonia. Endocrinol Nutr. 2015;62:210–6.
32. Van Caenegem E, Wierckx K, Taes Y, et al. Body composition, bone turnover, and bone mass in trans men during testosterone treatment: 1-year follow-up data from a prospective case-controlled study (ENIGI). Eur J Endocrinol. 2015;172:163–71.
33. Deplewski D, Rosenfiled R. Role of hormones in pilosebaceous unit development. Endocr Rev. 2000;21:363–92.
34. Ebling FJ, Skinner J. The measurements of sebum production in rats treated with T and oestradiol. Br J Dermatol. 1967;79:386–93.

35. Baldassarre M, Giannone FA, Foschini MP, et al. Effects of long-term high dose testosterone administration on vaginal epithelium structure and estrogen receptor-α and -β expression of young women. Int J Impot Res. 2013;25:172–7.
36. Schlatterer K, Von Werder K, Stalla GK. Multistep treatment concept of transsexual patients. Exp Clin Endocrinol Diabetes. 1996;104(06):413–9.
37. Grynberg M, Fanchin R, Dubost G, et al. Histology of genital tract and breast tissue after long-term testosterone administration in a female-to-male transsexual population. Reprod Biomed Online. 2010;20:553–8.
38. Perrone AM, Cerpolini S, Maria Salfi NC, et al. Effect of long-term testosterone administration on the endometrium of female-to-male (FtM) transsexuals. J Sex Med. 2009;6:3193–200.
39. Finkle WD, Greenland S, Ridgeway GK, et al. Increased risk of non-fatal myocardial infarction following testosterone therapy prescription in men. PLoS One. 2014;9:e85805.
40. Elamin MB, Garcia MZ, Murad MH, Erwin PJ, Montori VM. Effect of sex steroid use on cardiovascular risk in transsexual individuals: a systematic review and meta-analyses. Clin Endocrinol (Oxf). 2010;72:1–10.
41. Olson-Kennedy J, Okonta V, Clark LF, et al. Physiologic response to gender affirming hormones among transgender youth. J Adolesc Health. 2017;62(4):397–401.
42. Fernandez JD, Tannock LR. Metabolic effects of hormone therapy in transgender patients. Endocr Pract. 2015;22(4):383–8.
43. Vita R, Settineri S, Liotta M, et al. Changes in hormonal and metabolic parameters in transgender subjects on cross-sex hormone therapy: a cohort study. Maturitas. 2018;107:92–6.
44. Cupisti S, Giltay EJ, Gooren LJ, et al. The impact of testosterone administration to female-to-male transsexuals on insulin resistance and lipid parameters compared with women with polycystic ovary syndrome. Fertil Steril. 2010;94(7):2647–53.
45. Chandra P, Basra SS, Chen TC, et al. Alterations in lipids and adipocyte hormones in female-to-male transsexuals. Int J Endocrinol. 2010;2010 [pii:945053].
46. Deutsch MB, Bhakri V, Kubicek K. Effects of cross-sex hormone treatment on transgender women and men. Obstet Gynecol. 2015;125(3):605–10.
47. Wultsch A, Kaufmann U, Ott J, et al. Profound changes in sex hormone levels during cross-sex hormone therapy of transsexuals do not alter serum cholesterol acceptor capacity. J Sex Med. 2015;12(6):1436–9.
48. Elbers JMH, Giltay EJ, Teerlink T, et al. Effects of sex steroids on components of the insulin resistance syndrome in transsexual subjects. Clin Endocrinol (Oxf). 2003;58(5):562–71.
49. Jacobeit JW, Gooren LJ, Schulte HM. Endocrinology: long-acting intramuscular testosterone undecanoate for treatment of female-to-male transgender individuals. J Sex Med. 2007;4(5):1479–84.
50. Jacobeit JW, Gooren LJ, Schulte HM. Safety aspects of 36 months of administration of long-acting intramuscular testosterone undecanoate for treatment of female-to-male transgender individuals. Eur J Endocrinol. 2009;161(5):795–8.
51. Maraka S, Singh Ospina N, Rodriguez-Gutierrez R, et al. Sex steroids and cardiovascular outcomes in transgender individuals: a systematic review and metaanalysis. J Clin Endocrinol Metab. 2017;102(11):3914–23.
52. Giltay EJ, Toorians AWFT, Sarabjitsingh AR, et al. Established risk factors for coronary heart disease are unrelated to androgen-induced baldness in female-tomale transsexuals. J Endocrinol. 2004;180(1):107–12.
53. Polderman KH, Gooren LJ, Asscheman H, et al. Induction of insulin resistance by androgens and estrogens. J Clin Endocrinol Metab. 1994;79(1):265–71.
54. Auer MK, Ebert T, Pietzner M, Defreyne J, Fuss J, Stalla GK, T'Sjoen G. Effects of sex hormone treatment on the metabolic syndrome in transgender individuals: focus on metabolic cytokines. J Clin Endocrinol Metab. 2018;103(2):790–802.
55. Toorians AW, Thomassen MC, Zweegman S, et al. Venous thrombosis and changes of hemostatic variables during cross-sex hormone treatment in transsexual people. J Clin Endocrinol Metab. 2003;88:5723–9.

56. Wierckx K, Mueller S, Weyers S, et al. Long-term evaluation of cross-sex hormone treatment in transsexual persons. J Sex Med. 2012;9:2641–51.
57. Ott J, Kaufmann U, Bentz EK, Huber JC, Tempfer CB. Incidence of thrombophilia and venous thrombosis in transsexuals under cross-sex hormone therapy. Fertil Steril. 2010;93:1267–72.
58. Wierckx K, Elaut E, Declercq E, et al. Prevalence of cardiovascular disease and cancer during cross-sex hormone therapy in a large cohort of trans persons: a case-control study. Eur J Endocrinol. 2013;169:471–8.
59. Bird D, Vowles K, Anthony PP. Spontaneous rupture of a liver cell adenoma after long term methyltestosterone: report of a case successfully treated by emergency right hepatic lobectomy. Br J Surg. 1979;66(3):212–3.
60. Westaby D, Paradinas FJ, Ogle SJ, et al. Liver damage from long-term methyltestosterone. Lancet. 1977;310(8032):261–3.
61. Sorelle JA, Jiao R, Gao E, Veazey J, Frame I, Quinn AM, Day P, Pagels P, Gimpel N, Patel K. Impact of hormone therapy on laboratory values in transgender patients. Clin Chem. 2019;65(1):170–9.
62. Singh-Ospina N, Maraka S, Rodriguez-Gutierrez R, et al. Effect of sex steroids on the bone health of transgender individuals: a systematic review and metaanalysis. J Clin Endocrinol Metab. 2017;102(11):3904–13.
63. Van Caenegem E, Wierckx K, Taes Y, et al. Bone mass, bone geometry, and body composition in female-to-male transsexual persons after long-term cross-sex hormonal therapy. J Clin Endocrinol Metab. 2012;97(7):2503–11.
64. Miyajima T, Kim YT, Oda H. A study of changes in bone metabolism in cases of gender identity disorder. J Bone Miner Metab. 2012;30(4):468–73.
65. Goh HHV, Ratnam SS. Effects of hormone deficiency, androgen therapy and calcium supplementation on bone mineral density in female transsexuals. Maturitas. 1997;26(1):45–52.
66. Van Kesteren P, Lips P, Gooren LJG, et al. Long-term follow-up of bone mineral density and bone metabolism in transsexuals treated with cross-sex hormones. Clin Endocrinol (Oxf). 1998;48(3):347–54.
67. Slagter MH, Gooren LJ, Scorilas A, Petraki CD, Diamandis EP. Effects of long-term androgen administration on breast tissue of female-to-male transsexuals. J Histochem Cytochem. 2006;54:905–10.
68. Stone JP, Hartley RL, Temple-Oberle C. Breast cancer in transgender patients: a systematic review. Part 2: female to male. Eur J Surg Oncol. 2018;44:1463–8.
69. Nikolic DV, Djordjevic ML, Granic M, et al. Importance of revealing a rare case of breast cancer in a female to male transsexual after bilateral mastectomy. World J Surg Oncol. 2012;10(1):280.
70. Burcombe RJ, Makris A, Pittam M, et al. Breast cancer after bilateral subcutaneous mastectomy in a female-to-male trans-sexual. Breast. 2003;12(4):290–3.
71. Shao T, Grossbard ML, Klein P. Breast cancer in female-to-male transsexuals: two cases with a review of physiology and management. Clin Breast Cancer. 2011;11(6):417–9.
72. Gooren L, Bowers M, Lips P, et al. Five new cases of breast cancer in transsexual persons. Andrologia. 2015;47(10):1202–5.
73. Van Renterghem SMJ, Van Dorpe J, Monstrey SJ, et al. Routine histopathological examination after female-to-male gender-confirming mastectomy. Br J Surg. 2018;105(7):885–92.
74. Urban RR, Teng NNH, Kapp DS. Gynecologic malignancies in female-to-male transgender patients: the need of original gender surveillance. Am J Obstet Gynecol. 2011;204(5):e9–12.
75. Dria'k D, Samudovsky M. Could a man be affected with carcinoma of cervix?- The first case of cervical carcinoma in trans-sexual person (FtM)-case report. Acta Medica (Hradec Kralove). 2005;48(1):53.
76. Taylor ET, Bryson MK. Cancer's margins: trans* and gender nonconforming people's access to knowledge, experiences of cancer health, and decision-making. LGBT Health. 2016;3(1):79–89.

77. Brown B, Poteat T, Marg L, Galea JT. Human papillomavirus-related cancer surveillance, prevention, and screening among transgender men and women: neglected populations at high risk. LGBT Health. 2017;4(5):315–9.
78. Futterweit W. Endocrine therapy of transsexualism and potential complications of long-term treatment. Arch Sex Behav. 1998;27(2):209–26.
79. Dizon DS, Tejada-Berges T, Koelliker S, et al. Ovarian cancer associated with testosterone supplementation in a female-to-male transsexual patient. Gynecol Obstet Invest. 2006;62(4):226–8.
80. Hage JJ, Dekker J, Karim RB, et al. Ovarian cancer in female-to-male transsexuals: report of two cases. Gynecol Oncol. 2000;76(3):413–5.
81. Clements-Nolle K, Marx R, Katz M. Attempted suicide among transgender persons: the influence of gender-based discrimination and victimization. J Homosex. 2006;51(3):53–69.
82. Bockting WO, Miner MH, Swinburne Romine RE, et al. Stigma, mental health, and resilience in an online sample of the US transgender population. Am J Public Health. 2013;103(5):943–51.
83. Budge SL, Adelson JL, Howard KAS. Anxiety and depression in transgender individuals: the roles of transition status, loss, social support, and coping. J Consult Clin Psychol. 2013;81(3):545.
84. Witcomb GL, Bouman WP, Claes L, et al. Levels of depression in transgender people and its predictors: results of a large matched control study with transgender people accessing clinical services. J Affect Disord. 2018;235:308–15.
85. Defreyne J, Kreukels B, T'Sjoen G, Staphorsius A, Den Heijer M, Heylens G, Elaut E. No correlation between serum testosterone levels and state-level anger intensity in transgender people: results from the European Network for the Investigation of Gender Incongruence. Horm Behav. 2019;110:29–39.
86. Asscheman H, Giltay EJ, Megens JA, de Ronde WP, van Trotsenburg MA, Gooren LJ. A long-term follow-up study of mortality in transsexuals receiving treatment with cross-sex hormones. Eur J Endocrinol. 2011;164:635–42.
87. Dhejne C, Lichtenstein P, Boman M, Johansson AL, Langstrom N, Landen M. Long-term follow-up of transsexual persons undergoing sex reassignment surgery: cohort study in Sweden. PLoS One. 2011;6:e16885.
88. Murad MH, Elamin MB, Garcia MZ, et al. Hormonal therapy and sex reassignment: a systematic review and meta-analysis of quality of life and psychosocial outcomes. Clin Endocrinol (Oxf). 2010;72(2):214–31.
89. Defreyne J, Motmans J, T'Sjoen G. Healthcare costs and quality of life outcomes following gender affirming surgery in trans men: a review. Expert Rev Pharmacoecon Outcomes Res. 2017;17(6):543–56.
90. Kuhn A, Bodmer C, Stadlmayr W, et al. Quality of life 15 years after sex reassignment surgery for transsexualism. Fertil Steril. 2009;92(5):1685–1689.e3.

Chapter 10
Testosterone as a Performance Enhancer

O. Hasan, M. Houlihan, D. Yang, and T. Kohler

10.1 Introduction

An interesting dichotomy is taking place: the world continues to decline in overall health fitness while there is a societal pressure, likely exacerbated by social media platforms, to achieve unrealistic patterns of body performance and physique. Supraphysiologic use of exogenous hormone replacement is allowing users to greatly increase muscle strength and athletic performance, often well beyond the limit attainable by natural causes [1]. As a result, more young people are taking exogenous testosterone for improved performance, quick results, and instant gratification. Derivatives of synthetic exogenous testosterone, anabolic androgenic steroids (AAS), were first introduced to athletes in the 1950s; however, it was not until the 1980s when the world started to notice abuse outside of the sports industry. AAS are a family of hormones that contain the natural hormone testosterone in addition to its close synthetic relatives [2]. They exhibit both "muscle building" (anabolic) and "masculinizing" (androgenic) properties, affecting a wide range of physiological systems [3]. While the term "steroids" is used with liberty to describe performance-enhancing drugs (PEDs), it should not be confused with steroids such as corticosteroids, which lack any anabolic potential and offer little abuse potential. Over the last 20–30 years, illicit AAS use has become a widespread phenomenon in the world [4–9]. As a result, it has become the subject of a vast literature of clinical and behavioral studies, too extensive to cover in its entirety. Therefore, this chapter primarily focuses on the illicit use of synthetic testosterone as a performance enhancer. We discuss the history and evolution of AAS in the last few decades and

O. Hasan
Cook County Health, Chicago, IL, USA

M. Houlihan · D. Yang · T. Kohler (✉)
Mayo Clinic, Rochester, MN, USA
e-mail: Kohler.Tobias@mayo.edu

© Springer Nature Switzerland AG 2021
J. P. Mulhall et al. (eds.), *Controversies in Testosterone Deficiency*,
https://doi.org/10.1007/978-3-030-77111-9_10

review current literature on the side effect profile of supraphysiologic use of AAS. Lastly, we discuss the evolving landscape of selective AAS, called selective androgen receptor modulators (SARMS) as hormone replacement.

10.2   Historical Context of Steroids/Hormone Replacement for Performance

Testosterone was first isolated in the 1930s [10, 11]. Numerous testosterone derivatives, we now call AAS, were soon synthesized. While these were largely prescribed to treat male hypogonadism, AAS were also being prescribed to treat depression in psychiatric patients as a possible cure for the "male climacteric" [10, 11]. AAS first received world prominence when the Soviet team was allegedly found to be using AAS at the 1954 Vienna weightlifting championships [12, 13]. AAS usage soon spread within competition bodybuilding, strength sports, and track and field events, where performance depended on muscle strength and faster recovery [14]. By the 1960s, its perceived performance-enhancing effect resulted in it being banned in the Olympics. However, throughout the 1960s and 1970s, AAS remained confined to higher levels of sport where its efficacy was a well-kept secret. Ironically, the medical community at the time claimed that AAS were ineffective for gaining muscle mass [13, 15, 16]. The American College of Sport Medicine famously issued a statement in 1977 claiming that AAS were not effective for muscle gains, only to later retract the statement in 1987 and indicate that AAS were indeed effective [17].

By the late 1970s and 1980s, competitive bodybuilding gained in popularity. AAS began to break out of the elite athletic community and into the general population who took idols such as Arnold Schwarzenegger [18]. Fitness and bodybuilding magazines bearing AAS-using male models on the front covers started to fill the shelves and bookbags of young adults. Young men were soon aware of the dramatic muscle gains that were now achievable with the use of AAS [19]. These were largely fueled by a series of underground guides of using AAS, beginning with Daniel Duchaine's *Original Underground Steroid Handbook*, and later with multiple revised editions [20–23]. This book soon became the bible in the bodybuilding world, offering detailed advice on types of AAS to use, self-instructions to inject, recommended dosages, and side effects [22, 23]. Similar guides, such as the Phillips' *Anabolic Reference Guide*, appeared in 1985 [24]. As these guides became readily available, thousands of young men began using AAS.

Another catalyst for the increasing popularity of AAS use was the reformed Western cultural emphasis on male muscularity [19]. Muscular male images started to flood Western movies, dramas, advertisements, magazines, and comic strips [24, 25]. Even men in *Playgirl* magazine became more muscular [24, 25]. Action toys, such as GI Joe in the United States and Action Man in the British Commonwealth, showed a steady increase in muscularity from normal action figures in the 1960s to markedly muscular bodies in the following decades [26]. The message was clear – muscularity was the new measure of male masculinity. Therefore, the climate was ripe for AAS to flourish in its appeal. Young men started to emulate the images they saw around them [27].

In the late 1980s, epidemiological studies started to document trends in AAS usage among young boys and men. Early studies showed that 6.6% of 3403 male 12th-grade students surveyed by anonymous questionnaires had used AAS at some time [28]. A third of the respondents stated that it was for "social" purposes rather than athletic performance. Another study conducted via questionnaire from the Monitoring the Future Study found that 3.0% of 12th-grade students of both sexes reported lifetime AAS use [4]. It was not until the 1990s that the US passed the Steroid Trafficking Act and soon designated AAS as schedule III-controlled substances [29, 30]. In 2004, the Anabolic Steroid Control Act amended the Controlled Substances Act and expanded its definition of anabolic steroids [30].

10.3   Current Trends in Steroid Abuse

Most of the AAS that athletes and non-athletes used were readily available as prescription drugs until more rigorous law enforcement began in 1991. Soon after, various AAS became available with the advent of the internet and over the counter as unregulated nutritional supplements. Today, various avenues are available to obtain AAS such as from "that guy" at a gym, dealers, or internet purchases [18]. Per one expert commentary, common reasons people take steroids are to look good in social settings, attract potential partners, or improve athletic performance in college or high school [18]. The commentary continues that police officers, prison guards, firemen, and military personnel are taking AAS to be bigger and stronger and to accomplish their objectives [18, 31]. AAS use is not unique to men, as lifetime prevalence rates of AAS use in women are 1.6%, possibly spurred on by the popularity of certain fitness trends such as CrossFit and others [32].

Arguably, the three most common methods of AAS administration are orally, transdermally, or by IM injection, the most popular of which is IM [30]. Illicit AAS users commonly structure their doses by employing two processes, "stacking" and "pyramiding," to maximize the anabolic effects. Stacking refers to taking two or more different steroids either by mixing agents or through varied routes [33]. This may entail receiving a total dose equivalent to 600–1000 mg per week, and in some cases, reportedly as high as 3000–5000 mg per week [34–36]. These latter doses are 50–100× the natural levels of testosterone production in a week [37]. Stacking may also involve a combination of both steroidal and non-steroidal derivatives with the latter providing concomitant anabolic effects (human Growth Hormone (hGH), Insulin-like Growth Factor (IGF) -1, and insulin). To counteract the negative side effects of AAS, other agents such as aromatase inhibitors, human chorionic gonadotropin, and estrogen receptor agonists/antagonists are also often used to maintain or stimulate endogenous testosterone production. Additionally, non-hormonal medications may be used to stimulate fat and water loss (diuretics and thyroid hormones) and to reduce the risk of detection (diuretics and probenecid) [27, 38]. Pyramiding, on the other hand, involves starting with a low dose and slowly increasing the dosages of different steroids. Cycles may be conducted over several weeks (4–12 weeks), followed by an off cycle of an additional 4–12 weeks [12, 39]. Using these approaches, some bodybuilders have reported AAS utilization of more than 1000 times the clinically recommended dosages for conditions such as hypogonadism [40]. At these levels, gains of up to 10 lbs of muscle have been reported in 1 month. The regimen of AAS in these settings is highly variable, with Table 10.1 summarizing AAS administration, pharmacokinetics, and costs [18].

Table 10.1 General overview of common substances abused to gain muscle

Agent	Route	Dose	Commonly reported purpose[a]	Beg.	Adv.	Other[a]
Dianabol	PO	2–3 pills/day	Mass builder and strength	X	2X	Originally formulated for POWS
Nandrolone decanoate	IM	2/week	Muscle building without water retention (no estradiol conversion)	X	3X	
Testosterone enanthate	IM	1/week	Raise T to recover faster and absorb more protein	X	3–4X	This and cypionate interchangeable
Testosterone cypionate	IM	1/week	Raise T to recover faster and absorb more protein		3–4x	This or enanthate picked for less H_2O retention
Winstrol	PO/IM	QOD inj	Strength builder – hardened look without water retention		X	Used by Olympic athletes and sprinters
Masteron	IM	QOD inj	Leaning and hardening agent		X	Favored by competitive bodybuilders
T3 (Cytomel)	PO	20 mcg +	Weight loss		X	
Clomiphene citrate	PO	25–50 mg/qod-qd	Take for 2–4 weeks immediately after cycle		X	Post-cycle therapy to prevent testis atrophy
Clenbuterol	PO	20 mcg+	B3 inhibitor to optimize muscle contraction		X	
Arimidex	PO	0.5–1 mg qod/qd	Used for gynecomastia or water retention		X	
IGF-1	IM	4–10 IU/day			X	Very expensive
Lasix/thiazides	PO	Few pills ×2 days			X	Used primarily for competitions
hCG	SubQ	2500 IU 2/week ×2 weeks	Take 2–4 weeks immediately after cycle		X	Also PCT – restores natural T production

Adv. advanced regimen, *Beg.* beginner regimen, *IM* intramuscular, *POWS* prisoners of war, *PCT* post-cycle therapy, *PO* by mouth – orally, *QD* every day, *QOD* every other day.
[a]Anecdotal report from an experienced AAS user [18] – comments are not validated and do not reflect views of the scientific community.

10.4   Mechanism of Performance Enhancement

The mechanism by which testosterone improves performance is not fully known. It is known that testosterone increases skeletal muscle mass by increasing myogenic differentiation of muscle progenitor cells which contribute to muscle fiber hypertrophy of type 1 and type 2 fibers [41–43]. Testosterone is further known to increase maximal voluntary strength and leg power while not impacting specific force [44]. It promotes mitochondrial biogenesis and increases net oxygen delivery by increasing red cell mass and promoting angiogenesis. Interestingly, testosterone also improves neuromuscular transmission and upregulates acetylcholinesterase expression in a frog hind limb model [45, 46]. There is speculation that this may reduce reaction time and therefore lead to better performance in sprint events and sports like baseball which requires a high level of hand-eye-coordination [30]. Testosterone may also impact mood and motivation, indirectly affecting athletic performance. Behavior effects of testosterone occurred within minutes in animal models with rats showing increased aggression and locomotion [47]. German scientists invented an androgen nasal spray that enhanced competitiveness without systemic effects [48]. There is speculation that these rapid actions of testosterone contributed to Floyd Landis' dramatic comeback on the mountainous stage of Tour de France [49].

10.5   Anecdotal Revelations of a Steroid Abuse Expert

The senior author's former patient, Chad Schaive, provides unique insight into the world of steroid abuse [18]. Although anecdotal, many of his insights are intuitive, and, as demonstrated later in the chapter, there is a dearth of quality information about supraphysiologic testosterone level effects. For example, Chad avoided testicular atrophy and problems with fertility through the collective knowledge of steroid abusers with use of clomiphene citrate and hCG several years prior to publications describing this practice [50–52].

Chad began abusing steroids early in life after he had success with natural weight training and working in a gym. He has successfully competed internationally in bodybuilding and powerlifting competitions and has had many experienced steroid abuse mentors and clients. Chad originally presented to the senior author's clinic after he abruptly quit testosterone and several other supplements upon the sudden death of his father. Some of the more thought-provoking insights Chad had to offer centered around what he perceived as the true risks of steroid abuse are and the lifestyle which accompanied.

Simple internet searches on premature deaths of professional wrestlers and bodybuilders reveal disturbing trends. When analyzing the death rates of previous professional wrestlers (i.e., high AAS users) who participated in Wrestlemania

128 O. Hasan et al.

events between 1985 and 2011, total death rates from cardiovascular disease, acute drug intoxications, and cancer were 35.5%, 17.8%, and 8.8%, respectively [53]. Chad speculated this was mainly due to the lifestyle affiliated with being a wrestler. People willing to inject steroids will often have no qualms about taking narcotics to combat pain from working out or use other more dangerous and addictive drugs. This point is well illustrated by "Goldman's Dilemma," a Faustian bargain developed by Dr. Robert Goldman in the 1980s, which trades guaranteed victory in competition from a drug in exchange for guaranteed death within 5 years. Relative acceptance of this bargain that was initially sensationally reported as >50% was formally tested in an online survey [54]. However, of 212 participants, only 1% accepted the initial terms of the bargain, whereas 6% would accept the bargain if the theoretical drug were legal. Interestingly, only 12% state they would use the illegal drug if there was no death condition.

At the same time, Chad stated that many AAS users recognize a finite human boundary, where those who reach 400 pounds from weightlifting often die prematurely from cardiac problems. A 2016 article titled "Big Dead Bodybuilders" supports this belief, listing out 31 dead bodybuilders who died between the ages 22 and 53, almost all of which died from cardiac etiologies. Renal based complications were cited as the cause of death in the remainder [55]. Another study revealed that national football league (NFL) defensive linemen had higher mortality related to cardiovascular disease than any other positions despite adjusting for playing time and body mass index, suggesting an association between significant muscle mass (AAS use) and mortality [56]. This association is further supported by other studies which reported AAS use in approximately 14.8% of NFL defensive linemen [57].

Chad further described other risks of steroid abuse including back spasms from dehydration, erectile dysfunction, testicular atrophy, acne, and balding. Additionally, he indicated that many AAS users experience a new set-point of normalcy, whereby they adjust to supraphysiologic testosterone levels and the associated stronger erections, higher energy, and greater sense of well-being. Inversely, the drop of testosterone to normal levels is often then associated with feelings of depression, suboptimal erections, reduced energy, and overall loss of a sense of well-being. He continues by stating that gains with high testosterone levels also create unrealistic expectations for users and their social circles. As one uses more and more steroids, cost may also become a problem. Many AAS abusers will have to take second jobs (security, personal training) to help support their habit. Others will turn to crime, become steroid dealers themselves, or resort to prostitution to help support their habit.

Ultimately, Chad counseled against AAS use. He recognized the appeal of the quick gains steroids can offer, but contended these can be achieved naturally and more sustainably with proper nutrition and consistent exercise.

10.6   Review of Literature on Supraphysiologic Testosterone Side Effects

The chronology mentioned in the evolution of AAS as PEDs has important implications in the evaluation of the long-term medical and psychiatric consequences of its use. It is significant to note that widespread illicit use of AAS did not occur among the general public until the 1980s and 1990s. As such, the majority of AAS users are younger and under 60 years of age [17]. The relatively young population has not reached an age of risk for diseases such as cardiovascular disease that occur later in life. As such, there is a deficiency in published literature commenting on long-term adverse side-effects. Only now will the long-term side effects begin to be visible in the aging population – a cohort that will be the first of its kind and spark a new wave of epidemiologic investigation. Adverse effects that have slowly begun to emerge and are of concern are categorized as cardiovascular, hematologic, psychiatric and neuropsychological, hormonal, and metabolic.

Cardiovascular Effects   In the last few decades, there have been multiple anecdotal reports of cardiovascular effects, such as hypertension [58, 59], dyslipidemia [60, 61], cardiomyopathy [62, 63], left ventricular hypertrophy [58, 64], myocardial ischemia [65–67], and arrhythmias [68, 69]. Larger, controlled studies more recently have supported these findings. AAS causing dyslipidemia is characterized by increased low-density lipoprotein and decreased high-density lipoprotein cholesterol, an established risk for atherosclerotic disease [60, 61]. One imaging study found higher calcium scores in long-term AAS weightlifters than men of comparable age [70]. Thiblin et al. conducted a postmortem study comparing 87 deceased men testing positive for AAS with 173 men in the control group. He found AAS users had greater cardiac mass after adjusting for age, body mass, and history of trauma [71]. Recent conduction studies have demonstrated abnormal tonic cardiac autonomic regulation [72], ventricular repolarization abnormalities [73], and decreased cardiac electrical stability in AAS users [74]. Akçakoyun et al. demonstrated increased intra- and inter-atrial electromechanical delay (AEMD) in healthy, young AAS-using bodybuilders, making them more prone to developing atrial fibrillation [75]. D'Andra et al. utilized cardiac echocardiogram studies to compare AAS-user athletes to non-AAS user athletes and non-athletes and found increased septal strain and decreased ventricular ejection fraction among AAS men [69]. It is important to note, however, that effects such as hypertension, dyslipidemia, and coagulation abnormalities may remit after AAS discontinuation, while loss of tissue elasticity and cardiomyopathy may be irreversible [76, 77].

Psychiatric Effects   Several field studies have described psychiatric symptoms associated with illicit AAS use. These suggested that some AAS users exhibit hypomanic or manic symptoms during AAS exposure, characterized by aggressiveness, exaggerated self-confidence, hyperactivity, reckless behavior irritability, and occasional psychotic symptoms [27, 78, 79]. Some studies showed depressive symptoms, characterized by loss of interest, anorexia, loss of libido, and occasional suicidality [39, 80, 81]. Other reports utilized personal interview and or psychological scales to compare AAS users with non-users. These psychiatric effects appear to be idiosyncratic with the majority of AAS users exhibiting minimal psychiatric symptoms and only a small minority exhibiting severe or disabling symptoms [82–85]. These differences can be partially attributable to differences in dosages or intervals of AAS use versus intervals of non-exposure, linking commonality of mood disorders with higher doses of AAS used, especially at levels >1000 mg per week [86–88]. Pagonis et al. assessed AAS use in two pairs of monozygotic twins and found that non-AAS-using twins showed no lifetime history of any psychopathology [89]. However, there is no clear causal role in AAS-induced psychiatric effects, and there appears to be significant variation in individual sensitivities to androgen excess, withdrawal, or deprivation [90, 91].

Occasional field studies have also documented cases of aggressive or violent behavior in some AAS users, with no history of violence or criminal behavior prior to AAS use. These behaviors include committed or attempted murder by previously normal individuals [92–94] or uncharacteristic violent or criminal behavior while using AAS [78]. In one study, 23 AAS users and 14 non-users were assessed regarding their relationships with wives and girlfriends [83]. Users reported more aggression toward women when using AAS than when not using AAS. While it is impossible to fully ascertain if AAS played a causal role in these various cases, it is important to note that individuals did not display similar behavior in the absence of AAS use. However, some authors argue that AAS are not causally linked to violence [95, 96]. Past users of AAS state that "roid rage" (feelings of aggressiveness, irritability, and anger) is overstated, citing that users are often on restrictive diets which adds to the overall irritability [18]. Manifestation of these behaviors may also stem from disproportionate steroid use in men with more aggressive and angry personalities at baseline [18].

Other Side Effects Some of the common side effects experienced by AAS users include back spasms (attributed to dehydration), testosterone "flu" from high-dose injections, erectile dysfunction, gynecomastia, balding, and acne [97]. Testicular atrophy/infertility was measured in one study as a form of regret by AAS users [98]. However, experienced AAS users often utilize combination hCG therapy for recovery of spermatogenesis and to avoid fertility issues [99]. For women, undesirable side effects include those of masculinization, including acne, hirsutism, and coarsening of voice [12]. Herlitz et al. assessed renal function in a cohort of 10 healthy bodybuilders after long-term AAS use. The bodybuilders experienced increased proteinuria (range 1.3–26.3 g/d) and renal insufficiency (serum creatinine range 1.3–7.8 mg/dl) with renal biopsy revealing focal segmental glomerulosclerosis in nine [100].

AAS use may also serve as a gateway to additional medications and drugs. Due to extensive exercise regimen, AAS users often suffer from chronic joint pain, which may lead to use of opiates [101]. In a study of 223 men entering a drug-rehab program, AAS use was higher among opioid users compared with men using other drugs [102]. Furthermore, about 30% of AAS users may develop dependence by a body image pathway or neuroendocrine pathway [103, 104]. A body image pathway refers to the observation that people start AAS due to preoccupation with their muscularity, referred to as muscle dysmorphia [105]. Neuroendocrine factors may contribute to AAS dependence by suppressing testosterone levels via negative feedback and resulting in hypogonadism upon discontinuation [106]. While some may minimize hypogonadism by supplementing clomiphene or hCG [107], many continue to display symptoms of hypogonadism for weeks or months. The feeling of fatigue, loss of libido, and depression may subsequently lead people to resume using AAS.

10.7   Future Trends in Steroid Abuse

Despite the new increasing literature on adverse effects of AAS, other factors limit the extent of research which may be conducted. One such factor is the inability to conduct controlled studies using AAS due to the long-term side effects. Most of the literature we have now is from field studies that are prone to selection and information biases. Another factor is the lack of trust among AAS users for physicians. Nearly 56% of AAS users surveyed in one study stated that they had never disclosed their AAS use to any physician [108]. It is important for current physicians to recognize this as a public-health concern as the bulk of the population who used AAS in the 1980s and 1990s are now reaching an age to display some of the long-term side effects discussed.

Lastly, performance-enhancing drugs are constantly evolving, and a new generation of drugs are emerging. SARMs are novel oral drugs which display tissue-specific activation of androgen signaling [109]. Androgen receptors are among a group of nuclear receptors which modulate DNA binding and transcription contingent on interaction with a ligand (i.e., testosterone) [110, 111]. SARM's mechanism of action can be both agonist and antagonist at the androgen receptor, with a high degree of selectivity for specific tissue receptors, thereby potentially minimizing the unintended side effects often seen with AAS [112]. The complexity of biochemical interaction of various SARMs with respective androgen receptors allows for the synthesis of a variety of SARMs which can perform antagonistic effects at desired tissue (e.g., prostate and seminal vesicles) while still enacting anabolic effects in skeletal muscle and bone [111]. Given the therapeutic benefit and pharmacokinetics of SARMs, they have been evaluated for utilization as a male contraception and for the treatment of benign prostatic hyperplasia, sexual dysfunction, osteoporosis, cachexia, muscular dystrophies, and Alzheimer's disease [113–119]. Testosterone, when utilized for performance enhancement, can induce potential untoward effects of erythrocytosis, peripheral aromatization of estrogen, hepatotoxicity, male pattern baldness, acne, diminished fertility, and serum lipid derangements [120]. In contrast, preliminary data from SARM studies suggest varied side-effect profiles. Additionally, SARMs are currently available as oral pharmacotherapeutic agents [121].

As a result of this targeted, efficacious therapeutic benefit of SARMs, they likely represent the next frontier in terms of pharmacotherapy for performance enhancement. Given their potential for abuse within the arena of athletic performance, the World Anti-doping Agency banned SARMs in athletic events [122]. Despite their relative scarcity as branded pharmacotherapy and lack of FDA approval, various SARMs are available for purchase online. Additionally, strength and conditioning websites and forums offer interested athletes "how-to" guides for optimal utilization of these understudied performance-enhancing drugs. Further study and evaluation of SARMs are necessary prior to demonstrating safety and efficacy for their medically intended purposes, let alone their utilization in the realm of performance enhancement.

10.8   Conclusions

Testosterone supplementation as a tool for performance enhancement dates back now roughly 70 years. The fierce nature of competition has motivated athletes and lay people alike to seek alternative avenues for physical development and competitive advantage. Evolving societal expectations regarding optimal male physique and masculinity have also played a role in the increased utilization of AAS among the general public. The physiologic impact of long-term AAS use is poorly understood at present; however, given the more common utilization of these medications in the 1980s and 1990s, the field is ripe for research on long-term impacts of these therapies. Although we are in an era which emphasizes evidence-based medicine, given the nature of AAS use, high-level data may not be available. Rather, transparent dialogue with patients interested in, currently using, and previously using AAS can educate providers and help optimize clinical knowledge and intervention. Just as a toxicologist benefits from understanding the patterns of patient's illicit drug abuse, so too can a provider learn from first-hand experience of patients using AAS. Optimal patient care, therefore, demands that clinicians understand the natural history of AAS use as a performance enhancer, thereby improving patient counseling and facilitating AAS cessation and recovery.

References

1. Kouri EM, Pope HG Jr, Katz DL, Oliva P. Fat-free mass index in users and nonusers of anabolic androgenic steroids. Clin J Sport Med. 1995;5:223–8.
2. Pope H, Brower K. Anabolic-androgenic steroid abuse. In: Sadock B, Sadock V, editors. Comprehensive textbook of psychiatry. Philadelphia: Lippincott Williams & Wilkins; 2005. p. 1318–28.

3. Sheffield-Moore M, Urban RJ. An overview of the endocrinology of skeletal muscle. Trends Endocrinol Metabol TEM. 2004;15:110–5.
4. Johnston LD, O'Malley PM, Bachman JG, Schulenberg JE. Volume II: College students and adults ages 19–45. Bethesda: National Institute on Drug Abuse; 2006. Monitoring the future national survey results on drug use, 1975–2005.
5. McCabe SE, Brower KJ, West BT, Nelson TF, Wechsler H. Trends in non-medical use of anabolic steroids by U.S. college students: results from four national surveys. Drug Alcohol Depend. 2007;90:243–51.
6. Galduroz JC, Noto AR, Nappo SA, Carlini EA. Household survey on drug abuse in Brazil: study involving the 107 major cities of the country--2001. Addict Behav. 2005;30:545–56.
7. Pallesen S, Josendal O, Johnsen BH, Larsen S, Molde H. Anabolic steroid use in high school students. Subst Use Misuse. 2006;41:1705–17.
8. Rachon D, Pokrywka L, Suchecka-Rachon K. Prevalence and risk factors of anabolic-androgenic steroids (AAS) abuse among adolescents and young adults in Poland. Sozial und Praventivmedizin. 2006;51:392–8.
9. Wanjek B, Rosendahl J, Strauss B, Gabriel HH. Doping, drugs and drug abuse among adolescents in the State of Thuringia (Germany): prevalence, knowledge and attitudes. Int J Sports Med. 2007;28:346–53.
10. David K, Dingemanse E, Freud J, Laquer E. Uber Krystallinisches mannliches Hormon Hoden (Testosteron), wirksamer als aus Harn oder aus Cholesterin Bereitetes Androsteron. Zeit Physiol Chem. 1935;233:281–2.
11. Wettstein A. Uber die kunstliche Herstellung des Testikelhormons Testosteron. Schweiz Med Wochenschr. 1935;16:912.
12. Borges T, Eisele G, Byrd C. Review of androgenic anabolic steroid use. Office of Safeguards and Security U.S. Department of Energy; 2001. p. 1–18.
13. Wade N. Anabolic steroids: doctors denounce them, but athletes aren't listening. Science. 1972;176:1399–403.
14. Fitzpatrick F. Where steroids were all the rage: a doctor's curiosity and a businessman's love of weightlifting set off a revolution in York. Philadelphia: Philadelphia Inquirer; 2002.
15. Casner SW Jr, Early RG, Carlson BR. Anabolic steroid effects on body composition in normal young men. J Sports Med Phys Fitness. 1971;11:98–103.
16. Haupt HA, Rovere GD. Anabolic steroids: a review of the literature. Am J Sports Med. 1984;12:469–84.
17. Kanayama G, Hudson JI, Pope HG Jr. Long-term psychiatric and medical consequences of anabolic androgenic steroid abuse: a looming public health concern? Drug Alcohol Depend. 2008;98:1–12.
18. Schaive C, Kohler TS. An inside perspective on anabolic steroid abuse. Transl Androl Urol. 2016;5(2):220–4. https://doi.org/10.21037/tau.2016.03.08.
19. Pope H, Phillips K, Olivardia R. The Adonis complex: the secret crisis of male body obsession. New York: Simon & Schuster; 2000a.
20. Duchaine D. The original underground steroid handbook; 1981.
21. Duchaine D. Underground steroid handbook; 1983.
22. Duchaine D. Underground steroid handbook II. Los Angeles: HLR Technical Books; 1989.
23. Phillips W. Anabolic reference guide. Golden: Mile High Publishing; 1985.
24. Leit RA, Gray JJ, Pope HG Jr. The media's representation of the ideal male body: a cause for muscle dysmorphia? Int J Eat Disord. 2002;31:334–8.
25. Leit RA, Pope HG Jr, Gray JJ. Cultural expectations of muscularity in men: the evolution of playgirl centerfolds. Int J Eat Disord. 2001;29:90–3.
26. Pope HG Jr, Olivardia R, Gruber A, Borowiecki J. Evolving ideals of male body image as seen through action toys. Int J Eat Disord. 1999;26:65–72.
27. Kanayama G, Hudson JI, Pope HG. Illicit anabolic-androgenic steroid use. Horm Behav. 2010;58(1):111–2.
28. Buckley WE, Yesalis CE 3rd, Friedl KE, Anderson WA, Streit AL, Wright JE. Estimated prevalence of anabolic steroid use among male high school seniors. JAMA. 1988;260:3441–5.

29. One Hundred First Congress. The Steroid Trafficking Act of 1990. Washington: U.S. Government Printing Office; 1990.
30. Pope HG Jr, Wood RI, Rogol A, Nyberg F, Bowers L, Bhasin S. Adverse health consequences of performance-enhancing drugs: an Endocrine Society scientific statement. Endocr Rev. 2014;35:341–75.
31. Second Report of the Senate Standing Committee (Chairman John Black). Drugs in sport. Canberra: AGPS; 1990. p. 357–68.
32. Sagoe D, Molde H, Andreassen CS, Torsheim T, Pallesen S. The global epidemiology of anabolic-androgenic steroid use: a meta-analysis and meta-regression analysis. Ann Epidemiol. 2014;24:383–98.
33. Brower KJ. Anabolic steroids. Psychiatr Clin North Am. 1993;16(3):97–103.
34. Fudala PJ, Weinrieb RM, Calarco JS, Kampman KM, Boardman C. An evaluation of anabolic-androgenic steroid abusers over a period of 1 year: seven case studies. Ann Clin Psychiatry. 2003;15:121–30.
35. Parkinson AB, Evans NA. Anabolic androgenic steroids: a survey of 500 users. Med Sci Sports Exerc. 2006;38:644–51.
36. Wilson-Fearon C, Parrott AC. Multiple drug use and dietary restraint in a Mr. Universe competitor: psychobiological effects. Percept Mot Skills. 1999;88:579–80.
37. Reyes-Fuentes A, Veldhuis JD. Neuroendocrine physiology of the normal male gonadal axis. Endocrinol Metab Clin North Am. 1993;22:93–124.
38. Hildebrandt T, Lai JK, Langenbucher JW, Schneider M, Yehuda R, Pfaff DW. The diagnostic dilemma of pathological appearance and performance enhancing drug use. Drug Alcohol Depend. 2011;114(1):1–11.
39. Pope HG Jr, Katz DL. Affective and psychotic symptoms associated with anabolic steroid use. Am J Psychiatry. 1988;145(4):487–90.
40. Dangle RD. Anabolic steroids. J Psychoactive Drugs. 1990;22:77–80.
41. Bhasin S, Woodhouse L, Casaburi R, et al. Testosterone dose-response relationships in healthy young men. Am J Physiol Endocrinol Metab. 2001;281(6):E1172–81.
42. Sinha-Hikim I, Artaza J, Woodhouse L, et al. Testosterone induced increase in muscle size in healthy young men is associated with muscle fiber hypertrophy. Am J Physiol Endocrinol Metab. 2002;283(1):E154–64.
43. Sinha-Hikim I, Roth SM, Lee MI, Bhasin S. Testosterone induced muscle hypertrophy is associated with an increase in satellite cell number in healthy, young men. Am J Physiol Endocrinol Metab. 2003;285(1):E197–205.
44. Storer TW, Magliano L, Woodhouse L, et al. Testosterone dose-dependently increases maximal voluntary strength and leg power, but does not affect fatigability or specific tension. J Clin Endocrinol Metab. 2003;88(4):1478–85.
45. Leslie M, Forger NG, Breedlove SM. Sexual dimorphism and androgen effects on spinal motoneurons innervating the rat flexor digitorum brevis. Brain Res. 1991;561(2):269–73.
46. Blanco CE, Popper P, Micevych P. Anabolic-androgenic steroid induced alterations in choline acetyltransferase messenger RNA levels of spinal cord motoneurons in the male rat. Neuroscience. 1997;78(3):873–82.
47. Clark AS, Henderson LP. Behavioral and physiological responses to anabolicandrogenic steroids. Neurosci Biobehav Rev. 2003;27(5):413–36.
48. Dickman S. East Germany: science in the disservice of the state. Science. 1991;254:26–7.
49. Walsh D. From lance to landis: inside the American doping controversy at the Tour de France. New York: Ballantine Books; 2007.
50. Coviello AD, Matsumoto AM, Bremner WJ, et al. Low-dose human chorionic gonadotropin maintains intratesticular testosterone in normal men with testosterone-induced gonadotropin suppression. J Clin Endocrinol Metab. 2005;90:2595–602.
51. Hsieh TC, Pastuszak AW, Hwang K, Lipshultz LI. Concomitant intramuscular human chorionic gonadotropin preserves spermatogenesis in men undergoing testosterone replacement therapy. J Urol. 2013;189:647–50.

52. Ramasamy R, Armstrong JM, Lipshultz LI. Preserving fertility in the hypogonadal patient: an update. Asian J Androl. 2015;17:197–200.
53. Herman CW, et al. The very high premature mortality rate among active professional wrestlers is primarily due to cardiovascular disease. Plos One. 2014;9(11):e109945. https://doi.org/10.1371/journal.pone.0109945.
54. Connor J, Woolf J, Mazanov J. Would they dope? Revisiting the Goldman dilemma. Br J Sports Med. 2013;47(11):697–700.
55. Collucci C. Big dead bodybuilders: the ultimate price of pro bodybuilding? 28 October 2016. Available: https://www.t-nation.com/pharma/big-dead-bodybuilders. Accessed 2019 Mar 30.
56. Baron SL, et al. Body mass index, playing position, race, and the cardiovascular mortality of retired professional football players. Am J Cardiol. 2011;109(6):889–96.
57. Horn S, Gregory P, Guskiewicz KM. Self-reported anabolic-androgenic steroids use and musculoskeletal injuries: findings from the Center for the Study of Retired Athletes Health Survey of Retired NFL Players. Am J Phys Med Rehabil. 2009;88:192–200.
58. Urhausen A, Albers T, Kindermann W. Are the cardiac effects of anabolic steroid abuse in strength athletes reversible? Heart. 2004;90:496–501.
59. Kuipers H, Wijnen JA, Hartgens F, Willems SM. Influence of anabolic steroids on body composition, blood pressure, lipid profile and liver functions in body builders. Int J Sports Med. 1991;12:413–8.
60. Bonetti A, Tirelli F, Catapano A, Dazzi D, Dei Cas A, Solito F, Ceda G, Reverberi C, Monica C, Pipitone S, Elia G, Spattini M, Magnati G. Side effects of anabolic androgenic steroids abuse. Int J Sports Med. 2007;29:679–87.
61. Hartgens F, Rietjens G, Keizer HA, Kuipers H, Wolffenbuttel BH. Effects of androgenic-anabolic steroids on apolipoproteins and lipoprotein (a). Br J Sports Med. 2004;38:253–9.
62. Vogt AM, Geyer H, Jahn L, Schänzer W, Kübler W. Cardiomyopathy associated with uncontrolled self medication of anabolic steroids [in German]. Z Kardiol. 2002;91(4):357–62.
63. Ferenchick GS. Association of steroid abuse with cardiomyopathy in athletes. Am J Med. 1991;91(5):562.
64. Payne JR, Kotwinski PJ, Montgomery HE. Cardiac effects of anabolic steroids. Heart. 2004;90:473–5.
65. Halvorsen S, Thorsby PM, Haug E. Acute myocardial infarction in a young man who had been using androgenic anabolic steroids [in Norwegian]. Tidsskr Nor Laegeforen. 2004;124(2):170–2.
66. Fineschi V, Baroldi G, Monciotti F, Reattelli LP, Turillazzi E. Anabolic steroid abuse and cardiac sudden death: a pathologic study. Arch Pathol Lab Med. 2001;125(2):253–5.
67. Kennedy C. Myocardial infarction in association with misuse of anabolic steroids. Ulster Med J. 1993;62(2):174–6.
68. Lau DH, Stiles MK, John B, Young GD, Sanders P. Atrial fibrillation and anabolic steroid abuse. Int J Cardiol. 2007;117(2):e86–7.
69. D'Andrea A, Caso P, Salerno G, Scarafile R, De Corato G, Mita C, Di Salvo G, Severino S, Cuomo S, Liccardo B, Esposito N, Calabro R, Giada F. Left ventricular early myocardial dysfunction after chronic misuse of anabolic androgenic steroids: a Doppler myocardial and strain imaging analysis. Br J Sports Med. 2007;41:149–55.
70. Santora LJ, Marin J, Vangrow J, et al. Coronary calcification in body builders using anabolic steroids. Prev Cardiol. 2006;9(4):198–201.
71. Far HR, Ågren G, Thiblin I. Cardiac hypertrophy in deceased users of anabolic androgenic steroids: an investigation of autopsy findings. Cardiovasc Pathol. 2012;21(4):312–6.
72. Maior AS, Carvalho AR, Marques-Neto SR, Menezes P, Soares PP, Nascimento JH. Cardiac autonomic dysfunction in anabolic steroid users. Scand J Med Sci Sports. 2013;23(5):548–55.
73. Maior AS, Menezes P, Pedrosa RC, Carvalho DP, Soares PP, Nascimento JH. Abnormal cardiac repolarization in anabolic androgenic steroid users carrying out submaximal exercise testing. Clin Exp Pharmacol Physiol. 2010;37(12):1129–33.

74. Sculthorpe N, Grace F, Jones P, Davies B. Evidence of altered cardiac electrophysiology following prolonged androgenic anabolic steroid use. Cardiovasc Toxicol. 2010;10(4):239–43.
75. Akcakoyun M, Alizade E, Gundogdu R, Bulut M, Tabakci MM, Acar G, et al. Long-term anabolic androgenic steroid use is associated with increased atrial electromechanical delay in male bodybuilders. Biomed Res Int. 2014;2014:451520.
76. Hartgens F, Kuipers H. Effects of androgenic-anabolic steroids in athletes. Sports Med. Auckland, NZ. 2004;34:513–54.
77. Rothman R, Weiner R, Pope H Jr, et al. Anabolic androgenic steroid induced myocardial toxicity: an evolving problem in an ageing population. BMJ Case Rep. 2011;pii:bcr0520114280.
78. Hall RC, Hall RC, Chapman MJ. Psychiatric complications of anabolic steroid abuse. Psychosomatics. 2005;46(4):285–90.
79. Talih F, Fattal O, Malone D Jr. Anabolic steroid abuse: psychiatric and physical costs. Cleve Clin J Med. 2007;74(5):341–344, 346, 349–352.
80. Parrott AC, Choi PY, Davies M. Anabolic steroid use by amateur athletes: effects upon psychological mood states. J Sports Med Phys Fitness. 1994;34(3):292–8.
81. Cooper CJ, Noakes TD, Dunne T, Lambert MI, Rochford K. A high prevalence of abnormal personality traits in chronic users of anabolic-androgenic steroids. Br J Sports Med. 1996;30(3):246–50.
82. Bahrke MS, Wright JE, Strauss RH, Catlin DH. Psychological moods and subjectively perceived behavioral and somatic changes accompanying anabolic-androgenic steroid use. Am J Sports Med. 1992;20(6):717–24.
83. Choi PY, Pope HG Jr. Violence toward women and illicit androgenic-anabolic steroid use. Ann Clin Psychiatry. 1994;6(1):21–5.
84. Midgley SJ, Heather N, Davies JB. Levels of aggression among a group of anabolic-androgenic steroid users. Med Sci Law. 2001;41(4):309–14.
85. Moss H, Panzak G, Tarter R. Personality, mood, and psychiatric symptoms among anabolic steroid users. Am J Addict. 1992;1:315–24.
86. Pagonis TA, Angelopoulos NV, Koukoulis GN, Hadjichristodoulou CS. Psychiatric side effects induced by supraphysiological doses of combinations of anabolic steroids correlate to the severity of abuse. Eur Psychiatry. 2006;21(8):551–62.
87. Pagonis TA, Angelopoulos NV, Koukoulis GN, Hadjichristodoulou CS, Toli PN. Psychiatric and hostility factors related to use of anabolic steroids in monozygotic twins. Eur Psychiatry. 2006;21(8):563–9.
88. Pope HG, Katz DL. Psychiatric effects of exogenous anabolic-androgenic steroids. In: Wolkowitz OM, Rothschild AJ, editors. Psychoneuroendocrinology: the scientific basis of clinical practice. Washington, DC: American Psychiatric Press; 2003. p. 331–58.
89. Pope HG, Brower KJ. Anabolic-androgenic steroid-related disorders. In: Sadock B, Sadock V, editors. Comprehensive textbook of psychiatry. 9th ed. Philadelphia: Lippincott Williams, Wilkins; 2009. p. 1419–31.
90. Daly RC, Su TP, Schmidt PJ, Pagliaro M, Pickar D, Rubinow DR. Neuroendocrine and behavioral effects of high dose anabolic steroid administration in male normal volunteers. Psychoneuroendocrinology. 2003;28(3):317–31.
91. Schmidt PJ, Berlin KL, Danaceau MA, et al. The effects of pharmacologically induced hypogonadism on mood in healthy men. Arch Gen Psychiatry. 2004;61(10):997–1004.
92. Choi PY, Parrott AC, Cowan D. High-dose anabolic steroids in strength athletes: effects upon hostility and aggression. Hum Psychopharmacol. 1990;5:349–56.
93. Pope HG Jr, Katz DL. Homicide and near-homicide by anabolic-androgenic steroids for strength training. Pharmacotherapy. 2011;31(8):757–66.
94. Conacher GN, Workman DG. Violent crime possibly associated with anabolic steroid use. Am J Psychiatry. 1989;146(5):679.
95. Klötz F, Petersson A, Isacson D, Thiblin I. Violent crime and substance abuse: a medico-legal comparison between deceased users of anabolic androgenic steroids and abusers of illicit drugs. Forensic Sci Int. 2007;173(1):57–63.

96. Klötz F, Petersson A, Hoffman O, Thiblin I. The significance of anabolic androgenic steroids in a Swedish prison population. Compr Psychiatry. 2010;51(3):312–8.
97. Kohler TS. Supra-physiologic testosterone supplementation: do body builders know something we don't? February 7, 2018. Accessed Mar 2020. https://grandroundsinurology.com/supra-physiologic-testosterone-supplementation-do-body-builders-know-something-we-dont/.
98. Kovac JR, Scovell J, Ramasamy R, Rajanahally S, Coward RM, Smith RP, Lipshultz LI. Men regret anabolic steroid use due to a lack of comprehension regarding the consequences on future fertility. Andrologia. 2015;47:872–8.
99. Wenker EP, Dupree JM, Langille GM, et al. The use of HCG-based combination therapy for recovery of spermatogenesis after testosterone use. J Sex Med. 2015;12:1334–7.
100. Herlitz LC, et al. Development of focal segmental glomerulosclerosis after anabolic steroid abuse. J Am Soc Nephrol. 2010;21(1):163–72.
101. Skarberg K, Nyberg F, Engstrom I. Multisubstance use as a feature of addiction to anabolic-androgenic steroids. Eur Addict Res. 2009;15(2):99–106.
102. Kanayama G, Cohane GH, Weiss RD, Pope HG. Past anabolic-androgenic steroid use among men admitted for substance abuse treatment: an underrecognized problem? J Clin Psychiatry. 2003;64(2):156–60.
103. Kanayama G, Barry S, Hudson JI, Pope HG Jr. Body image and attitudes toward male roles in anabolic-androgenic steroid users. Am J Psychiatry. 2006;163(4):697–703.
104. Kanayama G, Brower KJ, Wood RI, Hudson JI, Pope HG. Treatment of anabolic-androgenic steroid dependence: emerging evidence and its implications. Drug Alcohol Depend. 2010;109:6–13.
105. Pope HG Jr, Gruber AJ, Choi P, Olivardia R, Phillips KA. Muscle dysmorphia. An underrecognized form of body dysmorphic disorder. Psychosomatics. 1997;38(6):548–57.
106. Kashkin KB, Kleber HD. Hooked on hormones? An anabolic steroid addiction hypothesis. JAMA. 1989;262(22):3166–70.
107. Llewellyn W. Anabolics. 10th ed. Jupiter: Molecular Nutrition; 2011.
108. Pope HG, Kanayama G, Ionescu-Pioggia M, Hudson JI. Anabolic steroid users' attitudes towards physicians. Addiction. 2004;99(9):1189–94.
109. Narayanan R, Mohler ML, Bohl CE, Miller DD, Dalton JT. Selective androgen receptor modulators in preclinical and clinical development. Nucl Recept Signal. 2008;6:e010.
110. Chen J, Kim J, et al. Discovery and therapeutic promise of selective androgen receptor modulators. Mol Interv. 2005;5(3):173–88.
111. Miller CP, et al. Design, synthesis, and preclinical characterization of the selective androgen receptor modulator (SARM) RAD140. ACS Med Chem Lett. 2011;2(2):124–9.
112. Solomon ZJ, et al. Selective androgen receptor modulators: current knowledge and clinical applications. Sex Med Rev. 2019;7(1):84–94.
113. Chen J, Hwang DJ, et al. A selective androgen receptor modulator for hormonal male contraception. J Pharmacol Exp Ther. 2005;312(2):546–53. https://doi.org/10.1124/jpet.104.075424.
114. Ponnusamy S, et al. Androgen receptor agonists increase lean mass, improve cardiopulmonary functions and extend survival in preclinical models of Duchenne muscular dystrophy. Hum Mol Genet. 2017;26(13):2526–40. https://doi.org/10.1093/hmg/ddx150.
115. Vignozzi L, et al. Antiinflammatory effect of androgen receptor activation in human benign prostatic hyperplasia cells. J Endocrinol. 2012;214(1):31–43.
116. Watanabe K, et al. BA321, a novel carborane analog that binds to androgen and estrogen receptors, acts as a new selective androgen receptor modulator of bone in male mice. Biochem Biophys Res Commun. 2016;478(1):279–85.
117. Akita K, et al. A novel selective androgen receptor modulator, NEP28, is efficacious in muscle and brain without serious side effects on prostate. Eur J Pharmacol. 2013;720(1–3):107–14.

118. Miner JN, Chang W, Chapman MS, et al. An orally active selective androgen receptor modulator is efficacious on bone, muscle, and sex function with reduced impact on prostate. Endocrinology. 2007;148(1):363–73.
119. Jones A, et al. Effects of a novel selective androgen receptor modulator on dexamethasone-induced and hypogonadism-induced muscle atrophy. Endocrinology. 2010;151(8):3706–19.
120. Thirumalai A, et al. Treatment of hypogonadism: current and future therapies. F1000 Research. 2017;6:68.
121. Clark RV, et al. Safety, pharmacokinetics and pharmacological effects of the selective androgen receptor modulator, GSK2881078, in healthy men and postmenopausal women. Br J Clin Pharmacol. 2017;83(10):2179–94.
122. Thevis M, et al. Detection of the arylpropionamide-derived selective androgen receptor modulator (SARM) S-4 (andarine) in a black-market product. Drug Test Anal. 2009;1(8):387–92. https://doi.org/10.1002/dta.91.

Index

© Springer Nature Switzerland AG 2021
J. P. Mulhall et al. (eds.), *Controversies in Testosterone Deficiency*,
https://doi.org/10.1007/978-3-030-77111-9

Printed in the United States
by Baker & Taylor Publisher Services